THE CONCUSSION CRISIS IN SPORT

Concussion has become one of the most significant issues in contemporary sport. The life-changing impact of head injury and the possible threat that chronic traumatic encephalopathy poses to children and young athletes in particular is calling into question the long-term future of some of our most well-established sports. But what are the real issues behind the headlines and the public outcry, and what can and should be done to save sport from itself? This concise, provocative introduction draws on perspectives from sociology, medicine, ethics, psychology, and public health to answer these questions and more.

The book explores the context in which the current cultural crisis has emerged. It assesses the current state of biomedical knowledge; the ethics of regulating for brain injury; the contribution of the social sciences to understanding the behaviour of sports participants; and the impact of public health interventions and campaigns. Drawing on the latest research evidence, the book explores the social roots of sport's concussion crisis and assesses potential future solutions that might resolve this crisis.

This is essential reading for anybody with an interest in sport, from students and researchers to athletes, coaches, teachers, parents, policy-makers, and clinicians.

Dominic Malcolm is Reader in the Sociology of Sport at Loughborough University, UK. He is also Editor-in-Chief of the *International Review for the Sociology of Sport*.

THE CONCUSSION CRISIS IN SPORT

Dominic Malcolm

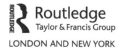
Routledge
Taylor & Francis Group

LONDON AND NEW YORK

First published 2020
by Routledge
2 Park Square, Milton Park, Abingdon, Oxon OX14 4RN

and by Routledge
52 Vanderbilt Avenue, New York, NY 10017

Routledge is an imprint of the Taylor & Francis Group, an informa business

British Library Cataloguing in Publication Data
A catalogue record for this book is available from the British Library

Library of Congress Cataloging-in-Publication Data
A catalog record has been requested for this book

ISBN: 978-0-367-26291-4 (hbk)
ISBN: 978-0-367-26293-8 (pbk)
ISBN: 978-0-429-29240-8 (ebk)

Typeset in Bembo
by Taylor & Francis Books

CONTENTS

TABLES

ABBREVIATIONS

AFL	Australian Football League
AfPE	Association for Physical Education
ALS	Amyotrophic Lateral Sclerosis
AMSSM	American Medical Society for Sports Medicine
BBBC	British Board of Boxing Control
CDC	Centers for Disease Control and Prevention
CISG	Concussion in Sport Group
CMOs	Chief Medical Officers
CTE	Chronic Traumatic Encephalopathy
FA	Football Association
FIELD	Football's Influence on Lifelong Health and Dementia Risk
FIFA	Fédération Internationale de Football Association
ICC	International Cricket Council
IIHF	International Ice Hockey Federation
IOC	International Olympic Committee
IRB	International Rugby Board
KT	knowledge transfer
MMA	mixed martial arts
mTBI	mild traumatic brain injury
mTBIC	Mild Traumatic Brain Injury Committee
NATA	National Athletic Trainers Association
NCAA	National Collegiate Athletic Association
NCPE	National Curriculum for Physical Education
NFL	National Football League
NHL	National Hockey League
NRL	National Rugby League
PAEG	Physical Activity Expert Group

PFA	Professional Footballers' Association
PTSD	Post-Traumatic Stress Disorder
RFL	Rugby Football League
RFU	Rugby Football Union
RTP	return-to-play
SCAT	Sport Concussion Assessment Tool
SCIC	Sport Collision Injury Collective
SIS	second impact syndrome
SRC	sport-related concussion
SRI	sports-related injury
UEFA	Union European de Football Associations
WHO	World Health Organization

1

INTRODUCTION

Ash lay on the pitch gradually coming to. There were voices all around giving contradictory advice. 'You'll be fine, see how you feel in 5 minutes'. Others were more cautious: 'take a break, it's not worth the risk'. Ash had been concussed before but now the voices were coming from all directions and getting louder and louder. Perhaps it was time to retire. 'Game over?'

Crisis is a big word. Consider the 2008–2009 financial crisis that saw the near collapse of the global banking system, the humanitarian crisis in Yemen in 2018 where an estimated 22 million people were in need of aid, or the Ebola health crisis which affected over 28,000 people across ten countries in 2014. But crisis is also a widely used word. On the day of writing this introduction, the British media used the word 'crisis' in relation to Brexit, recycling, the penal system, a bank's IT system, murder rates in Latin America, and the number of players injured at one football (soccer) club. Crisis is often used as a rhetorical device to generate interest. So, is *The Concussion Crisis in Sport* simply hype or does it refer to something more tangible?

Concussion is defined as 'a traumatic brain injury induced by biomechanical forces' which typically: 1) results from a direct blow to the body; 2) leads to 'the rapid onset of short-lived impairment of neurological function that resolves spontaneously'; and 3) entails 'functional disturbance rather than a structural injury' (McCrory et al. 2017: 1). But the concussion crisis is a rather broader phenomenon. Partly this is due to the imprecision of what is meant by concussion such that even the very appropriateness of the term 'concussion' is debated. Should we talk specifically about *sport-related* concussion (SRC) or are these simply part of the broader spectrum of 'brain injury' (Sharp and Jenkins 2015)? Some make the case for supplanting concussion with the term 'mild traumatic brain injury' (mTBI), while others argue that labelling such conditions as 'mild' provides a highly

5.   The concussion crisis entails us asking questions about pastimes and activities which we had not only taken for granted but thought were positively good for us. This introspection has led groups that were previously united in their support of sport to become divided. The fundamental discrepancy between expectations and achievements relates to whether the sport-health ideology – sport seen as fundamentally good for our physical and mental health, an essential part of avoiding a range or illnesses, and providing a unique contribution to building 'character' (Waddington 2000) – holds good, or whether participation ultimately destroys our cognitive abilities and thus the defining qualities of being human.

On these grounds, the title 'concussion crisis' seems warranted. We are clearly experiencing more than just an abnormal period in the development of sport, more than just a questioning of the status quo, and more than just the reassessment of certain value judgements about sport. We need to ask some wide-ranging and deeply probing questions if we are to better understand this acute social conflict that defines the crisis.

In addressing SRC as a crisis, I have explicitly rejected the idea that we are witnessing 'a public health *epidemic*' (Zemek et al. 2016: 1015; emphasis added. See also Marshall and Spencer 2001 and Carroll and Rosner 2011 for scientific and populist examples of this representation of concussion as an epidemic). I do so for three reasons. First, use of the term 'epidemic' suggests that concussion is rife or especially prevalent and, as we will see, there remains a debate about the degree to which the recorded increase in the incidence of concussion is attributable to changes in awareness, measurement, and investigation (see Chapter 4). Second, 'epidemic' can imply that a condition is catching, a position which is clearly false. In this respect, the use of the term 'epidemic' is part of the hype which positions the 'crisis' as out of human control and, therefore, like a natural disaster, compelling a united response. Third, 'epidemic' is essentially a biomedical term and as such is inappropriate for what – as I argue throughout the book – needs to be understood as a cultural phenomenon.

But as a cultural phenomenon, the study of crisis tells us something more broadly about the world in which we live. For instance, some have argued that the term crisis is such a widely used word today because our degree of interconnectedness as a global population, and the speed and variety of conventional and social media communications, 'creates' the perception that crisis is a more-or-less ever-present state of affairs (Bauman 2000; Beck 2008). While *The Concussion Crisis in Sport* does not centrally address this question, it does inevitably tell us something beyond the crisis itself, and poses fundamental questions about the societies we form. In what kind of society do questions about the consequences of head injuries incurred while playing sport become so especially significant that a cultural crisis develops?

The aims of *The Concussion Crisis in Sport* are therefore to explore the various dimensions of SRC as an issue and to identify the distinct features of certain contemporary societies that have led these concerns to come to the fore. The first of these aims requires a distinctly multidisciplinary approach, and the book explores a wide range of evidence and interrogates a number of different perspectives. In Chapter 4 we look at the biomedical evidence in relation to concussion (and related conditions), providing a state-of-the-art review and reflecting on what and how much is currently known. Subsequently, in Chapter 5, we consider the distinct ethical considerations in relation to regulating head injuries in sport, before exploring in Chapter 6 what behavioural science has shown us about the lived experience of concussion. Chapter 7 begins our synthesis of divergent bodies of knowledge as we look at the convergence of biomedical evidence, ethical implications and the realities of human behaviour. These intersect in public health debates and interventions in relation to concussion. This provides the ideal segue to Chapter 8, which provides a more concentrated focus on the second aim of *The Concussion Crisis in Sport*. Here we develop our understanding of concussion in relation to a set of wider social processes, looking at the relationship between medicine, health, risk, ageing, commercialization, nationalism, celebrity, and violence (amongst others) in contemporary societies, attempting to understand the social roots of concerns over SRC. In Chapter 9 we consider the future of sport's concussion crisis and the potential for resolution.

Before embarking on that analysis though, we need to look in more detail about what the concussion crisis entails and how it came to be. Therefore, in the next two chapters we look at how head injury in sport became a social issue and the multiple ways in which the issue now permeates various spheres of social life. The aim here is to demonstrate how tangible is the crisis related to concussion in contemporary sport.

References

Bauman, Z. (2000) *Liquid Modernity*. Cambridge: Polity Press.

Beck, U. (2008) *World at Risk*. Cambridge: Polity Press (2nd Edition).

Cantu, R. and Hyman, M. (2012) *Concussions and Our Kids*. Boston, MA: Mariner Books.

Carroll, L. and Rosner, D. (2011) *The Concussion Crisis: Anatomy of a Silent Epidemic*. New York: Simon and Schuster.

Fainaru, S. and Fainaru-Wada, M. (2019) 'For the NFL and all of football, a new threat: an evaporating insurance market', 17 January, www.espn.co.uk/espn/story/_/id/25776964/insurance-market-football-evaporating-causing-major-threat-nfl-pop-warner-colleges-espn

Fraas, M. and Burchiel, J. (2016) 'A systematic review of education programmes to prevent concussion in rugby union', *European Journal of Sport Science*, 16(8): 1212–1218.

Fry, J. (2017) 'Two kinds of brain injury in sport', *Sport, Ethics and Philosophy*, 11(3): 294–306.

Greenhow, A. and Gowthorp, L. (2017) 'Head injuries and concussion issues', in N. Shulenkorf and S. Frawley (eds.), *Critical Issues in Global Sports Management*, Abingdon, UK: Routledge, 93–112.

Holton, R. (1987) 'The idea of crisis in modern society', *The British Journal of Sociology*, 38(4): 502–520.

Hruby, P. (2019) 'As the SuperBowl approaches, is high school football dying a slow death?', *The Guardian*, 30 January, www.theguardian.com/sport/2019/jan/30/high-school-football-numbers-drop-brain-trauma

Marshall, S. and Spencer, R. (2001) 'Concussion in rugby: the hidden epidemic', *Journal of Athletic Training*, 36(3): 334–338.

McCrory, P., Meeuwisse, W., Dvorak, J. et al. (2017) 'Consensus statement on concussion in sport: the 5th international conference on concussion in sport held in Berlin, October 2016', *British Journal of Sports Medicine*, 51: 838–847.

McNamee, M. (2014) 'Professional football, concussion, and the obligation to protect head injured players', *Sport, Ethics and Philosophy*, 8(2): 113–115.

McPherson, B., Curtis, J., and Loy, J. (1989) 'Defining sport', in B.D. McPherson, J.E. Curtis and J.W. Loy (eds.), *The Social Significance of Sport*. Champaign, IL: Human Kinetics.

Rader, M. (1947) 'Toward a definition of cultural crisis', *The Kenyon Review*, 9(2): 262–278.

Sharp, D. and Jenkins, P. (2015) 'Concussion is confusing us all', *Practical Neurology*, 15: 172–186.

Waddington, I. (2000) *Sport, Health and Drugs: A Critical Sociological Perspective*. London: E&FN Spon.

Zemek, R., Barrowman, N., Freedman, S. et al. (2016) Clinical risk score for persistent postconcussion symptoms among children with acute concussion in the ED', *Journal of the American Medical Association*, 315(10): 1014–1025.

2

CONCUSSION AS A SOCIAL ISSUE

Having played for 30 years, Ash was no stranger to head injury. But things were different now. When Ash had started playing, all they needed was a cold sponge, but now you could sense the worry: the dangers of dementia, second impact syndrome, motor neuron disease, etc. What Ash had once thought was something only boxers experienced, now seemed to be happening across the world of sport. 'How has it come to this?'

How should we begin to understand social issues? The unpredictability of human life can sometimes mean that specific events thrust an issue into the limelight and make it impossible to ignore. More commonly, however, a cultural crisis will grow out of a fairly narrow set of concerns which eventually generates a debate which becomes so far reaching that ultimately the issue gains a place on broader social and political agendas. In such cases, tracing the development of social issues helps us to identify the most significant elements.

Equally, the question of *which* social issues come to dominate the public agenda is more than simply a consequence of their self-evident importance. Consider this: why does the crisis confronting sport focus on a particular *type* of sports-related injury (SRI) and not sports injuries in general? While SRIs are difficult to accurately quantify (Malcolm 2017), and do not generally feature as a public health concern (Finch 2012), the most comprehensive UK data we have shows that they are both significant in scale (amounting to approximately 30 million injuries per year) and cost (amounting to direct medical costs of treatment of £420m) (Nicholl et al. 1994; 1995). Estimates of the prevalence of SRC suffer from similar methodological issues but, indicatively, Mrazik et al. (2015) suggest that concussions amount to approximately 9 per cent of all SRIs, while Fraas and Burchiel (2016) note that within rugby union, where concussions are thought to be relatively frequent, estimates range from 4.5–25 per cent of all injuries (see Chapter 4 for a further discussion). We can see, therefore, that the absolute number of injuries is less important than their qualitative consideration for, as Partridge (2014: 65) notes, concussion 'seemingly generates more debate than all other sports injuries combined'.

To explain why, we need to understand the emergence of social issues in the context of power relations (Becker 1963), as the actions of socially influential people either promote or prevent such issues becoming part of a broader public agenda. Consequently, the next two chapters seek to substantiate the claim that sport has a concussion crisis by revealing the processes that led to and exemplify its contemporary manifestations. In Chapter 3 we look at what actions have been taken and how this is indicative of crisis, while here we focus on timing and ask, how did concussion *become* such an important social issue that it grew into a cultural crisis?

The genesis of concussion as a social issue

In 1624, a court trial found that Jasper Vinall died 'by misadventure and through his own carelessness' when he was hit on the head during a cricket match (Malcolm 2013). In 1822, essayist William Hazlitt described a prizefighter for whom, 'All traces of life, of natural expression, were gone from him. His face was like a human skull, a death's head, spouting blood. The eyes were filled with blood, the nose streamed blood, the mouth gaped blood' (cited in Sheard 2003: 25–6). In the late nineteenth century, GS Davies (founder of the prestigious Charterhouse School's museum) reflected on the football played during Victorian times, by saying that, 'hard knocks had to be taken cheerfully. A fierce charge was apt to send a player with his head against the wall and much skin was lost at times' (cited in Dunning and Sheard 2005: 49).

These selective accounts demonstrate two key points. First, there is nothing new about head injury incurred whilst playing sport. While there are different views on the first use of the term – Harrison (2014: 825) cites a definition of concussion dating from the mid-sixteenth century, while McCrory and Berkovic (2001) suggest a Persian physician called Razes used the term pre-AD 1000 – it is clearly a concern that has a long lineage. While there is a school of thought that sports have developed into more violent displays due to various modern developments (e.g. commercialization, training techniques that increase muscle mass and power), according to most historical accounts, contemporary sports are less injurious today than were their predecessors (Dunning 1999; see also Chapter 8). So while, as we will see in Chapter 4, research has revealed an increasing incidence of SRC in recent years, this is likely to be shaped both by: 1) the more extensive surveillance research undertaken; and 2) participants' changing attitudes and behaviours. Consequently, it may not be an increasing incidence of head injuries that has propelled concussion to social issue status in contemporary sport, but that issue status has led to the documentation of higher incidence rates.

The second point is that, historically, concern about head injury has largely been triggered by external appearances (i.e. blood). Consequently, we can see that the contemporary concussion crisis has entailed a qualitative shift in perceptions. Concerns have increasingly focussed on the subtler signs of brain dysfunction and, with them, concern about the potential longer-term effects. Indeed, many argue that invisibility is a unique characteristic of concussion. While that is something of an overstatement (see Chapter 6 for a discussion) the capacity of the lay person to visually 'diagnose' injury is an important consideration. In explaining the development of concussion as a social issue we therefore need to look at a combination of quantitative (apparent incidence) and qualitative (type of symptom manifested) dimensions of injury.

In terms of quantity, the high number of deaths in the association (or soccer) and rugby codes of football meant that these sports initially drew medical concern. From 1870, *The Lancet* waged a strong campaign against the dangers of soccer and listed annual death rates until numbers seemed to subside and the campaign was withdrawn in 1899. Concern here related not just to head injury but SRIs in general (Sheard 1998), and as the descriptions earlier in this section suggest, the distinction we now draw between fighting, collision and contact sports has not always been so less clear-cut.

Shortly after the *Lancet* campaign ended, studies of American college football began to document both the frequency of concussion and the potential for long-term behavioural consequences. Harvard team doctors recorded an incidence of almost one concussion per game during the 1906 season. The impact of such concerns was contained because visual evidence of damage and the evidential link between concussion and the subsequent 'insanity and alcoholism' that some claimed it entailed was largely missing. However, ultimately the mobilization of economic interests was more important than biomedical uncertainty in suppressing concerns. As financial interests in the game increased, colleges saw sport as an important recruitment tool and attempts were made to emphasize the capacity of football to develop important masculine qualities. Some evidence of the scale of harm was hidden, while technical 'solutions' such as enhanced protective equipment and improved playing technique came to the fore. Consequently, the public became convinced that the cost-benefit ratio of health risk relative to social good made the practice tolerable. What Harrison (2014) calls 'the first concussion crisis' was thus averted through the actions of socially powerful elites.

Boxing, however, while impacting on small numbers and supported by influential people, was vulnerable to critique because the activity essentially entailed the primary goal of disabling one's opponent by intentionally targeting the head, in seeking a 'knockout' (Loosemore et al. 2007). The health hazards of boxing were first mentioned in *The Lancet* in 1893, and at the turn of the century the journal sought to highlight concerns by publicising the death of three boxers. All had suffered head injuries – one never regained consciousness, while the other two suffered 'inter-cranial haemorrhage' and 'lacerations to the brain' – but various contributing factors were also identified, including over-excitement, anxiety and apoplexy, which seemed to detract from the dangers of boxing per se (Sheard 1998). However, a distinct shift occurred in 1928 when Harrison Martland introduced the term 'punch drunk' to describe ex-boxers who exhibited the symptoms of neurological deficit.

Martland could only speculate about the underlying damage, but the medical community's adoption of the term *dementia pugilistica* in 1937 shows how the ideas gained increasing acceptance (Castellani and Perry 2017). A British neurologist, Macdonald Critchley subsequently described how the changes developed over various timespans (from six to 40 years) and in 1957 introduced the term 'chronic progressive traumatic encephalopathy' to add a further layer of precision to the description of the condition (Shurley and Todd 2012).

Yet despite formal definition and what appeared to be compelling, if essentially only indicative, evidence of cerebral harm, many medical personnel continued to support boxing. Advocates downplayed the frequency of injury, stressed the dangers of other activities, continued to attribute injuries to other causes (like low intelligence or the contraction of syphilis), and present moral arguments about the character building properties of (amateur) boxing, and the relative dangers of boxing for money. Social and moral concerns were thus in many ways more significant than scientific debates in determining the fate of boxing (Sheard 1998) and this, as we will see, is a pattern repeated in the concussion crisis of the twenty-first century (see also Chapter 7 and Chapter 9).

The 1950s saw the more extensive medical regulation of the sport. In 1950 the European Boxing Union introduced a medical scheme for boxers and the British Board of Boxing Control (BBBC) established its first medical committee. In the following decade boxing organizations extended the compulsory medical examination of boxers (Welshman 1998). Critics, however, were not deterred. In 1952, two American sociologists estimated that 60 per cent of retired boxers were slightly punch drunk and 5 per cent severely so (Weinberg and Arond 1952). The first attempt to legally prohibit boxing in the UK was defeated in December 1960, but a second attempt in 1962 led to the commissioning of the so-called 'Roberts Report' which would be crucial in shifting the balance of medical opinion. Roberts studied a random sample of boxers and not only concluded that there were approximately 200 severely punch-drunk boxers in the UK, but correlated the incidence with career length and fight exposure (cited in Sheard 1998). In 1973, Corsellis and colleagues published an article which is now taken to be the first empirical proof of a consistent pattern of neurological changes in the brains of autopsied boxers (cited in Shurley and Todd 2012).

The growing medical evidence led to bans on *professional* boxing in communist Cuba and parts of Eastern Europe (partly due to an anti-capitalist critique), but also in Western Europe led by Iceland, Sweden, and Norway. The medical associations of Australia, Britain, and Canada, plus the World Medical Association, formally took oppositional stances to boxing around the 1980s, and from the 1990s there were legal prohibitions placed on the emerging variants of 'ultimate fighting' and mixed martial arts (MMA) in 40 US states (van Bottenburg and Heilbron 2006). Again, concerns did not solely relate to concussion, but injuries in the sport more generally. They were also clearly exacerbated by the apparent bloodshed and the depiction of the sport as 'no holds barred', suggesting a deregulated and 'barbaric' form of fighting.

Despite this opposition, libertarian ethical arguments against prohibition have been dominant (see Chapter 5), and bans on MMA and professional boxing have been rescinded in most countries (only in Iceland, Iran, Saudi Arabia, and North Korea does professional boxing remain prohibited).[1] Consequently, for almost 40 years there has been an essential stalemate between medical associations convinced of the dangers of boxing and in favour of a formal ban, and states reluctant to restrict individual liberty. What is different about the current concussion crisis in sport is that these quantitative and qualitative factors have combined, such that the concerns historically voiced about boxing have resurfaced in relation to a range of collision and contact sports in which there are far more, and more demographically diverse, participants. Paradoxically, however, the extension of these concerns has not been accompanied by such a medically unified call for prohibition.

The emergence of concussion as a contemporary social issue

The projection of these somewhat narrow and discrete concerns onto a much larger 'at risk' population began at the end of the twentieth century. At this time a report published by the National Health and Medical Research Council described the incidence of SRC as a public health concern in Australia's four football codes (cited in Greenhow 2018). In Europe a study of Norwegian ex-international footballers concluded that brain damage detectable through CT scans was attributable to multiple minor head impacts (Shurley and Todd 2012), while subsequently Italian researchers began discussing a seemingly heightened prevalence of amyotrophic lateral sclerosis (ALS) among retired professional soccer players. Also known as Lou Gehrig's disease after the New York Yankees baseball player who died from the condition in 1941, ALS is a form of motor neuron disease in which muscles progressively cease to function (the scientist Stephen Hawking being perhaps the most well-known person to have the condition). Except in a minority of genetically inherited cases, the cause of ALS is unknown, but a 2004 publication claimed that the prevalence of ALS among retired Italian footballers was at least 20 times higher than in the wider population (Piazza et al. 2004). A study published a year later concluded that the combination of statistically inflated prevalence, and evidence of a dose-response relationship (i.e. contracting ALS was linked to the degree of exposure to the sport), indicated 'that playing professional football is a strong risk factor for ALS' (Chiò et al. 2005: 472).

As with earlier indications of injuries amongst boxers, various potentially causal factors were identified. These included: legal or illegal therapeutic drugs use – Italian football was in the midst of an extensive enquiry into performance-enhancing drug use at the time (Malcolm and Smith 2015); absorption of the chemicals used to treat football pitches; excessive exercising; and repeated trauma from heading the ball. A follow-up study concluded that because inflated ALS incidence was not found in other sports (basketball and cycling) it could not be directly related to exercise per se (Chiò et al. 2009). The fact that some notable ex-players with ALS did not occupy playing positions that required a high frequency of heading cast further doubt over that causal connection. Concerns about the inflated incidence of ALS found amongst Italian footballers have not been replicated elsewhere even though a number of high profile cases in rugby union exist (most notably South Africa's Joost van der Westhuizen, Wales' Ken Waters, and Scotland's Doddie Weir).

But perhaps the most significant marker in this process was the death of Mike Webster in September 2002. Webster's long and successful career in the NFL had been based on a combative and resilient style of play, for one of the most notoriously combative and resilient NFL teams. He retired in 1990 but by the time he was inducted into the Hall of Fame in 1997 a steady cognitive decline was already apparent, and in 1999 the NFL awarded him disability benefits related to the brain trauma he experienced during his playing career. Webster's decline was intertwined with various health-harming behaviours, such as self-administering shots from a taser gun. He was also formally charged with fraudulently obtaining prescription medicines. While heart attack was identified as the cause of death, his obituary in *The New York Times* foregrounded the damage his head had sustained and effectively pre-empted the scientific discovery that was to follow:

> Mike Webster, whose Hall of Fame pro football career was followed by more than a decade of physical and psychological turmoil apparently brought on by repeated blows to the head on the field, died yesterday in a Pittsburgh hospital. He was 50.[2]

Thus, the narrative of Webster's sport-induced cognitive decline was already established (indeed Webster's physician had written 'chronic concussive brain injury' on the death certificate) (Carroll and Rosner 2011: 213), but Pittsburgh pathologist Bennet Omalu took the crucial step of seeking to substantiate this lay diagnosis and investigate Webster's condition in relation to *dementia pugilistica*. In order to establish a connection, he embarked on independent and self-financed tests from which he ultimately came to co-author a 2005 paper in *Neurosurgery* titled, 'Chronic Traumatic Encephalopathy in a National Football League Player'. By defining this as a new condition rather than a variant of *dementia pugilistica* or *chronic progressive traumatic encephalopathy* – both of which had existed for half a century – Omalu facilitated the broadening of the concussion agenda. This was a new condition specific, at this point in time, to American footballers. As in the case of boxing, the link between head injury, concussion, and longer-term neurological decline had a common sense logic, but ultimately it continued to rely on extrapolation rather than evidence of a causal link (even today, those who believe there to be a link, do so on the basis of common sense and the improbability that the emergent pattern could be attributed to anything else). But an important consequence of seeking to define a 'new' condition was the associated belief that collision and latterly contact sports held their own distinct risks.

The UK parallel of Mike Webster is Jeff Astle. Astle had played soccer for England and was renowned for his ability to head the ball. Astle, who later had a brief career as a television celebrity, began to exhibit the symptoms of dementia in the late 1990s at the age of 54. When Astle died in 2002, age 59, the coroner concluded that his dementia was due to the 'repeated minor trauma' of heading a football, and thus his death was decreed to have resulted from 'an industrial disease' (Slater 2017). An autopsy 12 years later diagnosed Astle as having CTE, thus opening up the possibility that 'sub-concussive' impacts rather than concussions per se may be the source of longer-term harm. Importantly, Astle has not been reported as experiencing psychological decline like the depression, self-harm, and uncharacteristic violence exhibited by Webster, but in the only Australian case of CTE (to date) – rugby union's Barry Taylor – such behavioural change appeared in parallel with the dementia-like symptoms of the condition.

Rather than the severity of symptoms, or numbers affected, the actions of individuals such as Omalu enabled SRC to achieve greater prominence as a social issue in America (as opposed to Italy or the UK). This was further helped by the campaigning of former footballer and professional wrestler Chris Nowinski and the writings of investigative journalist Alan Schwarz at *The New York Times*. Together they brought the potential link between the cases of ex-players' longer-term neurocognitive decline and the practices of elite sport to the attention of a broader public.[3] In 2007 Nowinski joined forces with Robert Cantu and established the Sports Legacy Institute (later the Concussion Legacy Foundation), 'dedicated to solving the concussion crisis by advancing the study, treatment and prevention of the effects of brain trauma in athletes and other at-risk groups'.[4] Nowinski and Cantu have since worked closely with the neuropathologist Ann McKee, who oversees the Boston University 'brain bank' to which many North American athletes' have donated or pledged to donate their brains for analysis.

While these individuals are perceived by many as 'champions' of this movement, the rising social pressures in relation to the prevalence of SRC evoked changes in athletes' behaviour that had somewhat equivocal consequences. First, as shown by the cases of Aaron Rodgers in the NFL in 2010, and Sidney Crosby in the National Hockey League (NHL) in 2011, (some) players started to act with more overt caution than had been evident in the past. The acts of these prominent players, who voluntarily and conspicuously withdrew themselves from games following head injury, raised awareness and sparked wider media debates and political pressures about the potential dangers of concussion (Anderson and Kian 2012; McGannon et al. 2013. See the section on cultural impact in Chapter 3).

Second, and conversely, concussion and related concerns about CTE were closely identified with a number of athlete suicides. In 2011, three NHL players died. Wade Belak's cause of death was unclear, but he had a history of depression that was frequently cited as a contributing factor. Rick Rypien had a similar clinical history and his death was determined as suicide. Derek Boogard was recovering from a concussion when he died from what was deemed to be an accidental drug and alcohol overdose. He was also subsequently diagnosed with CTE during autopsy. Also in 2011, an ex-NFL player, Dave Duerson, committed suicide by shooting himself in the chest. Junior Seau is believed to have taken his own life under similar circumstances a year later. Duerson's primary preoccupation appeared to be concerns over contracting CTE, as one of his final acts was to send text messages to his family requesting that his brain be analysed after his death (a diagnosis of CTE was later confirmed). NHL player Todd Ewen also took his own life in 2015, but a post-mortem showed no evidence to support his belief that he was developing CTE (Kuhn et al. 2017). The self-diagnosis of CTE has been replicated among soccer players in the UK and there has been widespread speculation over the incidence of dementia amongst members of England's 1966 World Cup winning soccer team but there has been no confirmed cases of CTE in this group and CTE has not been connected with any athlete suicides. One of the features which particularly compli-cates this issue/connection is the degree of overlap between the documented symp-toms of post-concussion, and the experience of retirement (depression, anxiety, isolation, and even suicidal ideation) (Caron et al. 2013).

A third feature of the concussion crisis, again seemingly distinctive to North America, has been the pre-emptive retirement of athletes. This trend started with Chris Borland, who in March 2015 retired as a San Francisco 49ers player at age 24 (Cassilo and Sanderson 2018). A number of other NFL players have followed. Borland was neither specifically medically advised to retire nor was suffering from a particular concussion incident, but he explicitly attributed his decision to concerns about the health risks associated with the game. The circularity of this debate – are psychological problems a manifestation of brain injury, or does concern about brain injury harm psychological well-being? – is an important fuel to the crisis.

While within North America research has progressively shown higher degrees of prevalence and earlier occurrences of neurocognitive impairment, globally con-sidered such cases have been relatively confined. Research at Boston University has detected evidence of CTE in 110 out of 111 deceased former NFL players (Mez et al. 2017), ten out of 16 former ice-hockey players,[5] and one athlete as young as 18.[6] In 2017, *Neurosurgery* published a paper claiming to have made the first diag-nosis of CTE in a living person (Omalu et al. 2018). In soccer, Patrick Grange was the first American and, at age 29, the youngest player to be diagnosed with CTE in 2012 (though he also had a pre-mortem diagnosis of ALS) but, since Jeff Astle, CTE has 'only' been diagnosed in one other named former professional footballer (Rod Taylor who died in April 2018). The evidence base is, however, growing and a study published in 2017 claimed that four former British footballers, taken from a sample of six who had already been diagnosed with Alzheimer's Disease, had been diagnosed with CTE post-mortem (Ling et al. 2017). Comparatively few rugby union or league players have been diagnosed with CTE – among the more notable cases are the aforementioned Barry Taylor, Ireland's Kenny Nuzum and New Zealand's Geoff Old. While no Australian rules footballer has been diagnosed with CTE, early findings from a UK study revealed that CTE had been found in around 75 per cent of former soccer and rugby players, compared to approximately 12 per cent of the general population.[7]

Consequently, we can see that while the spill-over effects of the concussion crisis are evident in an expanding range of sporting contexts, rather different concerns are expressed within and outside of North America. For instance, Partridge and

Hall (2014: 41) provide a series of quotes from Australian Football League (AFL), National Rugby League (NRL) and International Rugby Board (IRB) officials made in 2012 which effectively adopted what they call the 'we're not like the NFL' position to dismiss concerns about the relationship between sport participation and CTE. Consequently, in the absence of a continuing stream of post-mortem diagnoses of CTE, most major incidents in Europe and Australasia relate to players who have continued to play their respective sports while appearing to experience the symptoms of concussion. In rugby union, the Australian player George Smith was allowed to return to the pitch during the 2013 deciding 'test' against the British Lions, while concussion in soccer attracted global recognition when the German player Christoph Kramer similarly returned to the field during the Fédération Internationale de Football Association (FIFA) World Cup Final in Brazil in 2014. Across the various football codes, players such as Ryan Mason of Hull City FC, Shontayne Hape of Montpellier RUFC, Jonathon Brown of the Brisbane Lions AFC (three-time winner of the Robert Rose Award for the most courageous player) and Kat Merchant, who won the Rugby World Cup with England's women, are amongst the growing number of players who have retired from sport prematurely (though not pre-emptively) due to the on-going impact of concussion injuries. In field hockey, issues around concussion heightened when two of Great Britain's 2016 Olympic gold medalists – Shona McCallin and Nicola White – were forced to miss the 2018 World Cup due to ongoing symptoms. Finally, a small number of deaths due to head injury have also occurred. In November 2014, Australian cricketer Phillip Hughes died shortly after being hit by a cricket ball that struck him on the back of the head. In September 2018, a South African rugby union player, Kyle Barnes, died after a tackle left him with serious swelling to the brain. In early 2019, the media highlighted the deaths of four French rugby union players in eight months, two due to heart-related conditions and two due to brain injuries.[8] While the relationship between these individual cases and the broader dangers of concussion is to be established, it is characteristic of cultural crisis that so many and such varied cases fuel the perceptual divide.

But while the specifics of events differ between North America and elsewhere, we can see that a similar set of campaigning actors has emerged. Key in this regard has been the campaign undertaken by Peter Robinson highlighting the dangers of brain injury and concussion. Peter's 14-year-old son, Ben, died after being treated for head injuries three times during a school's rugby match in Northern Ireland in 2011. A subsequent hearing found that a doctor present at the game had not spotted the signs of concussion, and that the referee had been relatively inattentive to players' claims to being injured because he felt that some were being 'prima donnas and drama queens'.[9] A compelling feature of the story is that Ben's mother was present at the game, expressed concern about her son's health, but was told to 'calm down' when she attempted to intervene.[10] The coroner concluded that Ben had died from SIS (believed to be the first case in the UK) and in so doing stressed the importance of conservative concussion management. Similarly, Jeff Astle's daughter, Dawn, heads the Jeff Astle Foundation and its high-profile *Justice for Jeff* campaign which seeks to raise awareness of brain injury in sport, support independent research, and provide support to those living with dementia or neurological impairment.

Conclusion

This chapter has shown how, over the course of approximately 150 years, concern about the inherent violence of some sports has shifted to a more limited focus on just one of the myriad of SRIs people routinely experience. Moreover, in relation to this one injury type, a crisis has developed from a relatively narrow set of concerns about a discrete population participating in fighting sports, to all those who play in range a of collision and contact sports. We have further seen a growth in the range of sporting practices believed to lead to longer-term neuro-cognitive decline, from the forceful and purposeful disabling of the brain in boxing, to the frequent but (largely) unintentional head injury experienced by NFL and NHL players, and lower-level and more routine contact (e.g. heading in soccer) which occurs in the absence of any apparent symptoms of trauma. First identified as such in Australia in 1994, SRC and various related conditions is now firmly established as a serious public health concern across the US (Goldberg 2013) and most of the major English speaking nations of the world.

Despite many similarities we also see important and distinct cross-cultural manifestations of this crisis. Moreover, cross-fertilization of events in different nations is important in fuelling emergent concerns. But as the responses to the concussion crisis have varied significantly across the globe, in the next chapter we must explore the various actions that have been taken what has been the social response to this emergent social issue?

Notes

1 www.economist.com/news/international/21639526-more-countries-are-allowing-p rofessional-boxing-despite-risks-bouncing-back. Accessed 3 May 2018.
2 www.nytimes.com/2002/09/25/sports/mike-webster-50-dies-troubled-football-hall-of-famer.html. Accessed 6 June 2018.
3 For documentation of Schwarz's pioneering campaigning see www.nytimes.com/by/ala n-schwarz. Accessed 15 May 2018.
4 https://concussionfoundation.org/ Accessed 7 July 2018.
5 www.philly.com/philly/sports/flyers/eric-lindros-keith-primeau-cte-nhl-flyers-gary-bet tman-concussions-20180419.html Accessed 14 May 2018.
6 www.bu.edu/cte/our-research/case-studies/18-year-old/ Accessed 10 February 2019.
7 www.stuff.co.nz/sport/110041389/footballers-and-rugby-players-six-times-more-likely-to-have-degenerative-brain-disease–british-study Accessed 21 January 2019
8 www.independent.co.uk/sport/rugby/rugby-union/news-comment/nathan-soyeux-dea d-fourth-french-rugby-player-dies-nicolas-chauvin-france-a8721256.html Accessed 10 February 2019.
9 www.theguardian.com/sport/2013/dec/13/death-of-a-schoolboy-ben-robinson-concussion-rugby-union Accessed 15 May 2018.
10 'Health: concussion in sport,' *Hansard* Vol. 752, 27 February 2014. https://hansard.pa rliament.uk/Lords/2014-02-27/debates/14022788000224/HealthConcussionInSport Accessed 15 May 2018.

References

Anderson, E. and Kian, E. (2012) 'Examining media contestation of masculinity and head trauma in the National Football League', *Men & Masculinities*, 15(2): 152–173.

Becker, H.S. (1963) *The Outsiders*. New York: Free Press.

Caron, J., Bloom, G., Johnston, K., and Sabiston, C. (2013) 'Effects of multiple concussion on retired National Hockey League players', *Journal of Sport & Exercise Psychology*, 35: 168–179.

Carroll, L. and Rosner, D. (2011) *The Concussion Crisis: Anatomy of a Silent Epidemic*. New York: Simon and Schuster.

Cassilo, D. and Sanderson, J. (2018) '"I don't think it's worth the risk": media framing of the Chris Borland retirement in digital and print media', *Communication & Sport*, 6(1): 86–110.

Castellani, R. and Perry, G. (2017) 'Dementia pugilistica revisited', *Journal of Alzheimer's Disease*, 60(4): 1209–1221.

Chiò, A., Benzi, G., Dossena, M., Mutani, R., and Mora, G. (2005) 'Severely increased risk of amyotrophic lateral sclerosis among Italian professional football players', *Brain*, 128(3): 472–476.

Chiò, A., Calvo, A., Dossena, M., Ghiglione, P., Mutani, R., and Mora, G. (2009) 'ALS in Italian professional soccer players: the risk is still present and could be soccer-specific', *Amyotrophic Lateral Sclerosis*, 10(4): 205–209.

Dunning, E. (1999) *Sport Matters: Sociological Studies of Sport, Violence and Civilization*. London: Routledge.

Dunning, E. and Sheard, K. (2005) *Barbarians, Gentlemen and Players: A Sociological Study of the Development of Rugby Football*. Abingdon, UK: Routledge.

Finch, C. (2012) 'Getting sports injury prevention on to public health agendas: addressing the shortfalls in current information sources', *British Journal of Sports Medicine*, 46(1): 70–74.

Goldberg, D. (2013) 'Mild traumatic brain injury, the National Football League, and the manufacture of doubt: an ethical, legal, and historical analysis', *Journal of Legal Medicine*, 34(2): 157–191.

Greenhow, A. (2018) *Why the Brain Matters: Regulating Concussion in Australian Sport*. Unpublished PhD thesis, Monash University, Melbourne Australia.

Harrison, E. (2014) 'The first concussion crisis: head injury and evidence in early American football', *American Journal of Public Health*, 104(5): 822–833.

Kuhn, A., Yengo-Kahn, A., Kerr, Z., and Zuckerman, S. (2017) 'Sports concussion research, chronic traumatic encephalopathy and the media: repairing the disconnect,' *British Journal of Sports Medicine*, 51(24): 1732–1733.

Ling, H., Morris, H., Neal, J., Lees, A., Hardy, J., Holton, J., Revesz, T., and Williams, D. (2017) 'Mixed pathologies including chronic traumatic encephalopathy account for dementia in retired association football (soccer) players', *Acta Neuropathologica*, 133: 1–16.

Loosemore, M., Knowles, C., and Whyte, G. (2007) 'Amateur boxing and risk of chronic traumatic brain injury: systematic review of observational studies', *British Medical Journal*, 335: 809.

Malcolm, D. (2013) *Globalizing Cricket: Englishness, Empire and Identity*. London: Bloomsbury.

Malcolm, D. (2017) *Sport, Medicine and Health: The Medicalization of Sport?* London: Routledge.

Malcolm, D. and Smith, A. (2015) 'Football and performance enhancing drugs', in V. Møller, I. Waddington and J. Hoberman (eds.), *The Routledge Companion to Sport and Drugs*, London: Routledge, 103–114.

Martland, H.S. (1928) 'Punch drunk', *Journal of the American Medical Association*, 19: 1103–1107.

McCrory, P. and Berkovic, S. (2001) 'Concussion: the history of clinical and pathophysiological concepts and misconceptions', *Neurology*, 57: 2283–2289.

McGannon, K., Cunningham, S., and Schinke, R. (2013) 'Understanding concussion in socio-cultural context: a media analysis of a National Hockey League star's concussion', *Psychology of Sport and Exercise*, 14: 891–899.

Mez, J., Daneshvar, D.H., Kiernan, P.T. et al. (2017) 'Clinicopathological evaluation of chronic traumatic encephalopathy in players of American football', *Journal of the American Medical Association*, 318(4): 360–370.

Mrazik, M., Dennison, C., Brooks, B., Yeates, K.O., Babul, S., and Naidu, D. (2015) 'A qualitative review of sports concussion education: prime time for evidence-based knowledge translation', *British Journal of Sports Medicine*, 49: 1548–1553.

Nicholl, J.P., Coleman, P., and Brazier, J. (1994) 'Health and healthcare costs and benefits of exercise', *Pharmacoeconomics*, 5(2): 109–122.

Nicholl, J.P., Coleman, P., and Williams, B.T. (1995) 'The epidemiology of sports and exercise related injury in the United Kingdom', *British Journal of Sports Medicine*, 29(4): 232–238.

Omalu, B., DeKosky, S.T., Minster, R.L., Kamboh, M.I., Hamilton, R.L., and Wecht, C. H. (2005) 'Chronic traumatic encephalopathy in a National Football League player', *Neurosurgery*, 57(1): 128–134.

Omalu, B., Small, G., Bailes, J., Ercoli, L., Merrill, D., Wong, K.-P., Huang, S.-C., Satyamurthy, N., Hammers, J., Lee, J., Fitzsimmons, R., and Barrio, J. (2018) 'Postmortem autopsy-confirmation of antemortem [F-18]FDDNP-PET scans in a football player with chronic traumatic encephalopathy', *Neurosurgery*, 82(2): 237–246.

Partridge, B. (2014) 'Dazed and confused: sports medicine, conflicts of interest, and concussion management', *Bioethical Inquiry*, 11: 65–74.

Partridge, B. and Hall, W. (2014) 'Repeated head injuries in Australia's collision sports highlight ethical and evidential gaps in concussion management policies', *Neuroethics*, 8(1): 39–45.

Piazza, O., Sirén, A., and Ehrenreich, H. (2004) 'Soccer, neurotrauma and amyotrophic lateral sclerosis: is there a connection?', *Current Medical Research and Opinion*, 20(4): 505–508.

Sheard, K. (1998) '"Brutal and degrading": the medical profession and boxing, 1838–1984', *International Journal of the History of Sport*, 15(3): 74–102.

Sheard, K. (2003) 'Boxing in the western civilizing process', in E. Dunning, D. Malcolm, and I. Waddington (eds.), *Sport Histories: Figurational Studies of the Development of Modern Sports*, London: Routledge, 15–30.

Shurley, J. and Todd, J. (2012) 'Boxing lessons: an historical review of chronic head trauma in boxing and football', *Kinesiology Review*, 1: 170–184.

Slater, M. (2017) 'FA and PFA commission new study into risk of dementia from playing football', *The Independent*, November 23.

Van Bottenburg, M. and Heilbron, J. (2006) 'De-sportization of fighting contests: the origins and dynamics of no holds barred events and the theory of sportization', *International Review for the Sociology of Sport*, 41(3–4): 259–282.

Weinberg, S.K. and Arond, H. (1952) 'The occupational culture of the boxer', *American Journal of Sociology*, 62: 460–469.

Welshman, J. (1998) 'Only connect: the history of sport, medicine and society', *International Journal of the History of Sport*, 15(2): 1–21.

3

CONCUSSION AS A CULTURAL PHENOMENON

Ash arrived for pre-season training. All the talk was about the new law changes, what you could and couldn't do anymore, how referees and coaches would take you off if they were worried. Ash thought about the players in the news who had retired after head injury. Oh, and that film about the discovery of CTE. 'Concussion seems to be everywhere'.

The events described in the previous chapter portrayed two essential features of a cultural crisis: action and spill-over. Put differently, the intersection of multiple social events has culminated in a crisis over concussion in sport. But such is the nature of crisis, that this is not (or is no longer) *confined to* sport. Moreover, responses to the crisis vary across the globe and this lack of uniformity is illustrative of the continued imbalance within sporting communities and thus a crisis which is ongoing. Consequently, in this chapter we ask, what has been the cultural impact of the concussion crisis? We draw evidence from three main spheres: sport governance; politics and law; and popular culture. This analysis shows the ways in which sport's concussion crisis has impacted upon various aspects of contemporary society.

Sports governance

Within sports we can identify three main types of action that have been taken. Responses to concussion have mainly focussed on: changes to rules; expanded research programmes; and revised medical regulations, including more detailed advice to participants. Each of these is explored in turn.

Rule changes

The most obvious developments – to players and spectators at least – are changes to the rules of play that have been introduced in recent years. As this is an ongoing process, it is best to only identify the broad trends. Indicatively, various changes have been made to NFL regulations restricting specific tactics, player formations, and forms of contact (Casson et al. 2010). In 2010 the NFL began to radically increase the fines posed on players who were found guilty of illegal hits. Rugby union authorities have increasingly restricted the height of tackling and sought to reduce contact between airborne players, particularly where this may lead a player to fall head-first to the ground (although in 2019 the English RFU withdrew a trial intervention lowering the height of tackling when it was revealed that concussion rates appeared to be rising).[1] In ice hockey, the International Ice Hockey Federation (IIHF) has restricted tackling which includes body contact from particular directions (e.g. behind) and/or which is targeted at the head (McGannon et al. 2013). The AFL has revised its rules regarding 'bumping' (shoulder and hip contact designed to manoeuvre an opponent off the ball), and reduced front-on contact, or contact to the head, while lacrosse authorities have banned some types of contact (i.e. to the head) and police other plays more diligently. Soccer has been the most reluctant of all the sports caught up in the concussion crisis to implement changes to the way the game is played. FIFA's rules have not fundamentally changed, although in 2015 the US governing body prohibited under-11s from heading the ball, and restricted heading in training for 11–13-year-olds.[2] Ironically perhaps, combat sports such as boxing have not recently revised their rules to offer greater protection to the heads of participants.

Changes have also been implemented to training practices. The American Ivy League colleges have agreed to reduce full contact practices to two sessions per week during the season, and The Pop Warner League (junior American football) has similarly limited contact practices. The latter has also banned certain blocking and tackling drills (Cantu and Hyman 2012), and in 2016 announced plans to eliminate kick-offs in competitions for younger participants (Cassilo and Sanderson 2018). In Canadian ice hockey, body checking has been banned for players under 13 years old (Bullingham et al. 2017). As can be seen, these changes relate only to North American sport, but elsewhere rugby union has introduced training programmes for young rugby players designed to prevent player injuries (White et al. 2019).

Considerable attention has also been focused on technical solutions for protecting the head. The cricketing authorities in various countries have made the wearing of helmets compulsory for certain age groups and certain levels of play (e.g. in England compulsory helmet wearing was first introduced into age-grade cricket and eventually into professional cricket in 2016). Both in American football and cricket, efforts have focused on changing helmet design to provide greater protection (for instance, to the back of cricketers' heads, to prevent a repeat of the Philip Hughes fatality). Some ski resorts have introduced rules about mandatory helmet use (especially for children), while lacrosse authorities have been criticized for the inequity of having compulsory hard helmets for males but only compulsory eye protection for females.[3] Across sports, changes have been implemented despite the somewhat limited evidence that any of this equipment actually reduces the frequency or severity of head injury (see Chapter 4).

Research

Sports organizations have also been proactive in commissioning and funding research into concussion. The NFL was the first to do this, forming its Mild Traumatic Brain Injury Committee (mTBIC) in 1994 (Hardes 2017). In 1997 the NHL followed suit and established a Concussion Working Group. The work of the NFL's mTBIC was, however, to become extremely controversial when it was accused of working to effectively challenge and discredit research highlighting the potential dangers of concussion (Greenhow and Gowthorp 2017) and using its position of power to leverage favourable publication access in the journal *Neurology* (amounting to 16 articles). *Neurology's* editor-in-chief was Mike Apuzzo, who also acted as medical consultant to the New York Giants (see Fainaru-Wada and Fainaru 2013 for a discussion). The NFL has subsequently embarked on an extensive programme of research funding to address this legacy of distrust, for instance providing $60m to fund *The Head Health Challenge* programme focused on improving helmet design (Brayton et al. 2019).

While bodies such as the AFL, NRL, Union European de Football Associations (UEFA), and the Rugby Football Union (RFU) have all joined the NFL in implementing injury surveillance systems to chart the incidence, trends, and mechanisms of concussion injuries, more far reaching research studies are only just beginning to emerge outside of North America. For instance, in 2017 a joint FA/ Professional Footballers' Association (PFA) study was launched – Football's Influence on Lifelong Health and Dementia Risk, or FIELD – which will compare the physical and mental health of 15,000 former soccer players and 45,000 members of the public to assess whether the incidence of degenerative neurocognitive disease is more common in ex-professional players than the wider population (Gulland 2018). Also in 2017, the AFL agreed to allocate Aus$250,000 per year to concussion research as part of its collective bargaining settlement with players.[4] It has also commissioned a study to evaluate the impact of concussion guidelines and advice on the wider AFL-playing community.[5]

The concussion crisis has essentially compelled sports governing bodies to fund such research, with only the NHL explicitly bucking this trend and receiving significant criticism for failing to do so.[6] But decisions over specific research programmes create their own controversies. Criticisms have been voiced over the non-emergence of a proposed study of jockeys and CTE which was announced in 2016, and the AFL's interference with, and cancellation of, a research project it commissioned before it produced any meaningful results (Carlisle 2018). When World Rugby (the name of the rebranded International Rugby Board) publicized the findings of a 2015 study as providing no definitive links between rugby and long-term cognitive health issues, it was subsequently revealed that this conclusion had been extensively debated between the study's funder and its lead researcher (Patria Hume). It was revealed that the funder had restricted what results it would allow to be released, while Hume later described World Rugby's interpretation as 'irresponsible',[7] and subsequently published a journal article that concluded that 'past participation in rugby or a history of concussion were associated with small to moderate neurocognitive deficits . . . in athletes post retirement from competitive sport' (Hume et al. 2017: 1209). At the heart of these controversies are perceived conflicts of interest. While sports governing bodies appear obliged to fund research, critics have invariably questioned the parameters of these studies (do they ask the most significant questions?) and the motives of these organizations for doing so.

Revised medical regulations

To varying degrees each of the main sports affected have also adapted their concussion management practices. In line with medical consensus statements (see Chapter 4), there has been a movement towards introducing concussion exclusion rules (Partridge 2014); that is to say, policies which ensure that players diagnosed with concussion are immediately (and more consistently) removed from the field of play and are then restricted in terms of the speed with which they are allowed to return to play (RTP). Some sports recommend or even *require* elite players to undergo baseline cognitive testing to enable the more accurate diagnosis of concussion. While this is partly restricted due to cost, as if to underscore the American exceptionalism over concussion, in the US the Mayo Clinic offers free baseline testing to high school athletes in Arizona and Minnesota (Gilbert and Partridge 2012). Increasingly sports leagues like the NFL, the English (soccer) Premier League, and rugby union's Super Rugby 15 have: a) introduced independent concussion spotters (sometimes with access to video replay) to enable the identification of injured players; and b) required those diagnosed with concussion to be cleared to play by an independent expert rather than doctors employed by the player's own team (introduced, e.g., at the 2015 men's Rugby Union World Cup).

While the relatively unrestricted interchange of players in the NFL and NHL mean that player substitution is unproblematic the NRL, AFL, and World Rugby have each introduced additional substitution allowances in cases of concussion. By providing extra provision for the substitution of concussed players, teams are incentivized to take precautionary action because any impact on the team's performance will be (partly) mitigated. That such rule changes are contentious is evidenced by the case of Cricket Australia's implementation of a concussion substitution trial (somewhat distinct to cricket, substitutes can only be made for *injured* players and substitutes are prohibited from taking part in the more significant roles of batting, bowling, or wicketkeeping), which the International Cricket Council (ICC) would not allow them to extend to the elite domestic game or internationally. Rugby union has also introduced a head injury assessment protocol which provides clinicians with a longer time to diagnose concussion. The evidence to support the introduction of these changes is often very limited, and as we will see in Chapter 5, the ethical challenges are significant.

Indicative of the seriousness with which these regulatory changes have been implemented, such rulings are both extensive in nature and prominently placed in official documentation. For instance, the *Football Association Handbook* (2017–2018) contains five pages on medical regulations, about half of which directly pertain to concussion. The *RFL (Rugby Football League) Medical Standards* document contains six sections addressing medical personnel, data, equipment, anti-doping, miscellaneous policies, and finally, concussion, the latter of which extends to 23 pages. Australian cricket regulations include a 'Concussion and Head Trauma Policy' extending to nine pages, while the 'Concussion Policy' of England Hockey stretches to 13 pages. (Strangely, the *England Boxing Rule Book* (2018) contains no specific mention of concussion, but does list a series of medical suspensions to be imposed on boxers who have been 'knocked out' and/or suffered loss of consciousness.) The outcome of these distinct regulations is to position concussion as a unique injury (Partridge 2014).

All sports centrally affected have also implemented their own concussion awareness programmes to educate players, coaches, parents, etc. These may: rely on digital technology (like the Hockey Canada Concussion Awareness App); be aimed directly at the educational sector and children's behaviour (like the Sport and Recreation Alliance's Recognise, Remove, Recover, Return programme); be sport-specific (like the RugbySmart or BokSmart for New Zealand and South African rugby union respectively, SmartHockey in Canada, or the FA's 'If in doubt sit them out'); or be cross-sport national campaigns (such as the CDC's Heads Up resources). They may be on-going or have dedicated focal points (like USA Hockey's Team Up Day for concussion awareness). In New Zealand attendance at annual educational workshops is mandatory for all rugby union coaches and referees (Mrazik et al. 2015: 1550). The impact and debates around these educative and public health campaigns are explored in Chapter 7.

Political and legal interventions

Most of the world's larger English-speaking nations have also witnessed direct political involvement in sport's concussion crisis. The first and most significant was in the USA where two hearings of the Congress House of Judiciary Committee were initially held into 'Legal Issues Relating to Football Head Injuries'.[8] On 28 October 2009, the committee heard from medical practitioners and researchers, but notably *not* the head of the NFL's mTBIC, Ira Casson.[9] While the players' union was criticized for its slow response to the issue, the focus of questioning was NFL Commissioner Roger Goodell. The league was accused of neglect in protecting current players and in managing the cases of retired players who exhibited cognitive decline. Committee members argued that there was a history of denial and obfuscation by the NFL and compared the league's actions to those of 'big tobacco' when initially confronted with evidence that smoking caused lung cancer. Goodell was largely evasive, deferring to medical colleagues. When explicitly asked if there was a link between playing professional football and the likelihood of contracting a brain-related injury, he suggested that more research was needed, to the obvious irritation of Committee members. It has been argued that, in taking this stance, he 'consistently [stuck] to the program of establishing doubt and uncertainty' (Goldberg 2013: 175).

The fallout of the earlier hearing had seen Casson resign from his position on the NFL's mTBIC, but at the second hearing held on 4 January 2010 he continued to espouse the committee's historically held position that: 1) the link between sport and longer-term neurocognitive decline could only be evidenced in relation to boxing; 2) other factors such as drug use might be significant in NFL cases; and 3) the NFL's existing research programme would provide answers to the key outstanding issues. This came despite the fact that a month previous Greg Aiello, an NFL spokesperson, had publicly stated that, 'It's quite obvious from the medical research that's been done that concussions can lead to long-term problems'.[10] The NFL's formal position effectively changed in March 2016 when a league official appeared in front of a further Congressional hearing.

Subsequent Congressional inquiries have looked into a number of issues including, for example, the impact of concussion on high school athletes (20 May 2010), protecting school-age and student athletes (8 September 2010 and 23 Sept 2010 respectively), and youth sport concussion prevention and research (13 May 2016). In May 2014, President Barack Obama hosted the Healthy Kids and Safe Sports Concussion Summit at the White House, during which he called for more research and better awareness, talked of his own sporting experiences where he 'probably' had suffered 'mild' concussion (see Chapter 4 for a discussion of the meaningfulness of this term), and argued that a cultural shift was required to enact the level of change needed. He has also publicly stated that if he had a son, he would not want him to play professional football. Conversely, up until February 2019 (see Chapter 9), President Donald Trump's major statements on the issue revolved around complaints that the game has become overly protective, creating 'soft' players and therefore ruining the game.[11] In so doing he sought to appeal to those sectors of the population resentful of the influence of the liberal urban classes in America (Cassilo and Sanderson 2018).

The closest comparison to the US Congressional hearings has been in Ireland and the *Report on Concussion in Sport* produced by the Houses of Oireachtas Joint Committee on Health and Children in December 2014. The positioning of this as an explicitly child-focussed health issue rather than a critique of elite sport practices is in part a reflection of concussion-related events in Ireland, but continues the drift or spill-over effect of the crisis from elite to grassroots sport. Hearings were held with sports organizations, medical experts, and health practitioners to consolidate what was known about the risks to players and what protective measures could be taken to militate against concussion in sport. The notions of second impact syndrome (SIS) and the link with CTE were accepted as sufficiently evidenced to be taken as 'real' conditions, and the dissemination of what was deemed to be best practice to the broader sporting community (i.e. concussion management in elite sport) was identified as a priority. In contrast to American hearings, the committee chair explicitly remarked on the cooperative and receptive response from the sports community.[12]

UK politicians have similarly adopted a collaborative rather than adversarial approach with sports governing bodies. During a 2014 House of Lords debate, 'Health: Concussion in Sport,' the government was asked what concussion advice was being given to sports governing bodies and medical services. Contributors were critical of the tendency of ministers to defer to sports governing bodies on these issues (see Chapter 5 for a discussion of the rationale), and highlighted the need for better education of participants, implementation of existing tools, and training for family and emergency medical practitioners. Pleas were made for more effective liaison across relevant government departments – especially the departments of Health, Education (again emphasizing that this is a child-focussed issue), and Culture, Media, and Sport – and the establishment of a national concussion and head injury research centre (which has not occurred). Notably however, the government commended the work of both sports governing bodies and medical groups for 'tak[ing] this matter increasingly seriously', and developing head injury protocols.[13] Concussion-related issues were also prominent in Baroness Grey-Thompson's (2017) influential *Duty of Care in Sport* report.

Within the elected House of Commons, Chris Bryant MP has been particularly active. Initially he made speeches urging the rugby union authorities to be more proactive about concussion, and in 2018 he (re-)established an All-Party Parliamentary Group for Acquired Brain Injury to raise awareness and enhance access to rehabilitation services across the UK National Health Service. 'Education and concussion in sport' was one of four priority themes,[14] and following a meeting in May 2018, calls were made for 'fully integrated sports and government initiatives'.[15] In November 2018, Bryant had called for a unified set of protocols to apply at all levels of all sports across the UK,[16] a move that the Labour Party committed to adopt in its manifesto for the next General Election.[17]

The primary mechanism of political intervention, therefore, has been to put pressure on sports governing bodies rather than to enact legislation. Again, however, the US is the exception. The Lystedt Law, named after a young athlete who suffered life-altering injuries as a consequence of a SRC injury, was first introduced in Washington state and has since been adopted in part or in whole in all 50 US states.[18] The law has three parts: requiring the annual delivery of concussion education to players, parents, and coaches in all sports; the compulsory removal (and non-return) of concussed players; and clearance by a healthcare professional prior to re-commencing sports activities. However, it has been argued that the effectiveness of such legislation could be improved by a more *unified* approach and the imposition of penalties for noncompliance, and some have even criticized the wording of individual state laws for being 'deliberately vague' (Mrazik et al. 2015: 1553). In Canada, the Ontario provincial government has mandated that schools have concussion policies (Russell et al. 2017) and, following an inquiry into the death of Rowan Stringer, passed the Rowan's Law (Concussion Safety) Act which, while yet to be fully developed, is expected to become the Canadian equivalent of the aforementioned Lystedt Law (Greenhow 2018). Overall, therefore, legislation has been directed towards the control of children rather than adults (see Chapter 8).

In contrast to the apparent reluctance of states to legally intervene are the attempts of private individuals and groups to bring the concussion policies of sports governing bodies to legal account. In this respect FIFA, the National Collegiate Athletic Association (NCAA), the NHL and, most notoriously, the NFL have all been subject to litigation. For instance, US plaintiffs have accused FIFA of the mismanagement of concussion at junior levels, arguing that the governing body has failed to introduce appropriate steps to educate players and indeed continues to promulgate rules (e.g. permitting heading) which suggest that they have not fully embraced the risks inherent to the sport. The NCAA has similarly been charged with potentially mismanaging concussions, while a group of retired professional ice hockey players contend that the NHL failed in its duty of care by neither recognizing the degree of risks posed by concussion injuries nor implementing appropriate medical procedures. By comparison, while there have been a handful of Australian personal injury claims against sports organizations and criticisms voiced over the AFL's failure to ban 'bumping', there has been no case which has more fundamentally examined a governing body's negligence in relation to concussion (Greenhow and Gowthorp 2017). The situation in Ireland is similar, although the Dublin High Court did approve a €2.75m settlement against a high school and hospital judged to have been negligent in following return-to-play (RTP) protocols and providing treatment to a schoolboy who suffered serious head injury playing rugby (Anderson nd). In early 2019 a former English rugby union player prosecuted his former club doctor for failure to detect concussion and enact precautionary actions.

While some individual NFL teams have been sued by players, probably the most significant legal action to date was brought by retired NFL players against the league and, initially, the helmet manufacturer, Riddell Inc. What started as a suit filed in California in 2011 by 75 ex-players developed into a class action lawsuit incorporating over 300 players in 2014–2015. It was alleged that the NFL failed to discharge the duty of care it owed to its players because a conflict of interests (with wealth creation) led the league to conceal information emerging about the potential risks to players (Greenhow and Gowthorp 2017). Plaintiffs highlighted the league's glorification of violence in its public relations and media output as responsible for contributing to a culture of violence while at the same time denying the validity of initial research and publishing counter research in what has been described as a 'campaign to minimise the issue, by discrediting' (Greenhow and East 2015). The case concluded with an estimated $1bn settlement that came into effect in January 2017 and could implicate up to 20,000 retired players over a 65-year period. The NFL settled without accepting liability (and thus remains a highly emotive but still effectively unproven charge) and claimed to do so in the interests of not incurring unnecessary legal costs and prioritizing support for players' health (Greenhow and Gowthorp 2017). However, despite an explicit rejection of a link between head injury and any mood or behavioural symptoms (which were deemed both to be caused by various factors, and be so widespread in the population that they could not be directly associated with the sport), the hearing tacitly accepted that the link between playing the sport and CTE was sufficiently strong and would *eventually* be proven as and when diagnostic technology became more sophisticated (Hardes 2017). A group of around 30 former players are said to be planning a similar type of class action suit against the AFL,[19] and in a placatory move the AFL has agreed to commit Aus$4million per year to compensate players who experience career ending injury (albeit not limited to concussion).[20]

Cultural impact

The cultural impact of the concussion crisis in sport is dominated by the juxtaposition of the distressing tales of personal affliction (e.g. Mike Webster) we saw in Chapter 2, against the charge of corporate neglect (if not unethical behaviour) described in the previous section. While this combination has generated considerable popular interest, in terms of cultural impact, developments in North America have once again been more extensive, with a number of major film portrayals appearing in recent years. *Head Games* (2012) is a documentary developed by Chris Nowinski (as mentioned in Chapter 2), which explores evidence relating to the impact of concussion on the brain, the link with CTE, and especially the growing body of evidence about the implications for adolescent and female athletes. It was revised in 2014 and re-subtitled *The Global Concussion Crisis*. In similar vein, *The Last Gladiators* (2011) is a documentary focussing on the deaths of Boogaard, Rypien, and Belak, while *Gleason* (2016) charts the final five years of the life of New Orleans Saints footballer Steve Gleason who contracted ALS in 2011, focussing particularly on the player's physical decline and the impact on his family. *League of Denial* (2013) is a documentary portraying the death of Mike Webster, Bennett Omalu's initial 'discovery' of CTE, and subsequent attempts to have the condition recognized by both the scientific community and NFL administrators. Its initial broadcast drew an audience 50 per cent larger than the season average and a record number of visitors to the producer's website. The documentary is notable for its critique of the sport media's reproduction of the game's masculine values which serve to normalize the violence, injury, and attitudes that create and compound the harm done through concussion (including CTE). In so doing it forces attention onto the institutional practices, the 'economic, historical, cultural and political forces that are rarely part of public debate' (Furness 2016: 50). *Concussion* (2015) is a dramatization of effectively the same story but, due to the casting of major Hollywood star Will Smith in the role of Omalu, has probably had the most far-reaching and international cultural impact. By comparison a BBC documentary, *Dementia, Football and Me* (2017) is the primary UK film portrayal to date.

Three of these films (*Head Games, League of Denial*, and *Concussion*) have accompanying book accounts. But these texts form just the tip of an extensive body of literature exploring a wide range of perspectives on concussion. Among the hundreds of books about concussion listed on Amazon (although not all of these relate to sport) are scientific texts authored by neurologists and psychologists and accounts of leading practitioners and researchers such as Bob Cantu (Cantu and

argued that narratives are effectively structured to absolve the corporations of evoking a racialized discourse of black criminality which places responsibility with the decisions made by individual footballers (Brayton et al. 2018; Rugg 2019). Finally, some accounts have been critical of the 'overreliance on medico-scientific conceptions of CTE' which both ignore the current limitations in scientific knowledge and, in so doing, deflect attention away from the value of making cultural changes to reduce harm to participants (Ventresca 2018: 3). Indicatively, the establishment of the Boston 'brain bank' generates continued interest and parallel schemes in the UK and Australia. That *Time* magazine listed Ann McKee within its 100 most powerful people of 2018 shows the power of this narrative.

Conclusion

The aim of this chapter has been to illustrate how sport's concussion crisis has become a broad cultural phenomenon. Building on Chapter 2 which demonstrated 'when' and 'how' concussion became a social issue, this chapter has illustrated the 'what' – the responses of sports organizations, political and legal systems, and what might broadly be termed the cultural industries. It is important to note that none is simply a reflection of the others, for cultural crisis is fundamentally about the interdependence of various interests and groups. A spill-over effect can be seen, not just across sports, or different playing populations, but in terms of drawing more and more people from various backgrounds into debates about the action required for resolution. Thus, while a particularly notable finding from this review is that many of the more radical actions have been initiated in the US, it is clearly also the case that, despite a long legacy of American 'exceptionalism' in sport, events elsewhere in the world seem to be following North American concerns and fuelling momentum for change. Whereas for many years a hard and fast distinction was drawn between boxing (for which a relatively widely accepted body of evidence appeared to have been assembled) and all other sports, the boundaries between American football and various other collision and contact sports seem increasingly permeable.

Such cross-cultural and indeed temporal variation in the social response to concussion is perhaps to be expected, but one would expect greater uniformity or consistency between and amongst the academic researchers who like other interest groups have been drawn into these debates. In the next three chapters we explore what has been learnt about concussion in these scientific communities. We will examine the work of ethicists in debating the merits of various approaches and actions, and the findings of behavioural scientists in exploring the lived experience of concussion. But first, because concussion is primarily understood as a medical issue, and because medicine is such a powerful social institution, we start there. From a biomedical viewpoint, exactly what is and is not known in relation to sport and concussion?

Notes

1 www.bbc.co.uk/sport/rugby-union/47000468 Accessed 25 January 2019.
2 www.independent.co.uk/sport/football/news-and-comment/us-soccer-ban-heading-th
  e-ball-for-children-over-fears-of-concussion-and-head-injuries-a6728341.html. Accessed
  13 February 2016.
3 www.nytimes.com/2011/02/17/sports/17lacrosse.html?_r=0. Accessed 23 March 2016.
4 www.news.com.au/sport/afl/afl-to-fund-a-minimum-of-250000-a-year-for-concussion-re
  search/news-story/e95fe084d1bc8f9637acbf51ea00ea0b Accessed 25 January 2018.
5 www.aflcommunityclub.com.au/index.php?id=47&tx_ttnews%5Btt_news%5D=806&
  cHash=4cc7c4048b Accessed 25 January 2019.
6 www.nydailynews.com/sports/hockey/hbo-takes-aim-nhl-refusal-invest-cte-research-a
  rticle-1.3845018 Accessed 23 January 2018.
7 See www.worldrugby.org/news/81734?lang=en, www.bbc.co.uk/sport/rugby-union/
  33686163, and www.nzherald.co.nz/sport/news/article.cfm?c_id=4&objectid=11658681.
  Accessed 23 January 2019.
8 https://judiciary.house.gov/_files/hearings/printers/111th/111-82_53092.PDF Accessed
  15 January 2019.
9 www.nytimes.com/2009/10/29/sports/football/29hearing.html Accessed 8 March 2018.
10 www.nytimes.com/2010/01/05/sports/football/05concussions.html Accessed 8 March
   2018.
11 www.washingtonpost.com/gdpr-consent/?destination=%2fnews%2fmorning-mix%2fwp
   %2f2016%2f10%2f13%2ftrump-just-criticized-the-nfls-softer-rules-intended-to-help-pro
   tect-players-from-traumatic-brain-injury%2f%3f&utm_term=.9a287fbba564 Accessed 11
   January 2019.
12 https://webarchive.oireachtas.ie/parliament/media/joint-committee-on-health–childer
   e-report-on-concussion-in-sport1-171214.pdf Accessed 8 March 2018.
13 'Health: concussion in sport,' *Hansard* Vol. 752, 27 February 2014. https://hansard.pa
   rliament.uk/Lords/2014-02-27/debates/14022788000224/HealthConcussionInSport
   Accessed 8 March 2018.
14 www.nrtimes.co.uk/single-post/2018/01/26/Brain-injury-lobby-finds-its-voice Accessed 15 May 2018.
15 www.espn.co.uk/rugby/story/_/id/23441456/concussion-rfu-head-medicine-calls-grea
   ter-awareness-surrounding-head-injuries Accessed 8 May 2018.
16 www.bbc.co.uk/sport/46350379 Accessed 28 November 2018.
17 www.telegraph.co.uk/football/2018/11/26/labour-party-accuses-football-turning-blind
   -eye-concussion/ Accessed 28 November 2018
18 www.justice.org/state-concussion-laws Accessed 15 October 2018.
19 www.theage.com.au/sport/afl/winmar-considers-joining-concussion-class-action-2018
   0226-p4z1ts.html Accessed 15 October 2018.
20 www.news.com.au/sport/afl/afl-to-fund-a-minimum-of-250000-a-year-for-concussion
   -research/news-story/e95fe084d1bc8f9637acbf51ea00ea0b Accessed 17 February 2018.
21 This search of the Nexis was conducted on 1 May 2018. The following specific searches
   were undertaken: 'All UK national newspapers', 'Major US newspapers', 'Major Australian newspapers', 'All South African news sources', and 'News about Canada' were
   searched for 'sport and concussion or CTE'; 'Presse nationale France' was searched for
   'sport and commotion cérébrale or CTE'; and 'Publikationen aus Deutschland' (all news
   sources in German on Nexis) was searched for 'sport and konkussion or CTE'. Unfor-
   tunately it was not possible to search for New Zealand media content separately from
   Australia due to the way Nexis categorizes content.

References

Ahmed, O. and Hall, E. (2017) '"It was only a mild concussion": exploring the description of sports concussion in online news articles', *Physical Therapy in Sport*, 23(1): 7–13.

Anderson, E. and Kian, E. (2012) 'Examining media contestation of masculinity and head trauma in the National Football League', *Men & Masculinities*, 15(2): 152–173.

Anderson, J. (no date) 'Concussion, sport and the law', www.sportsintegrityinitiative.com/concussion-sport-and-the-law/

Benson, P. (2017) 'Big football: corporate social responsibility and the culture and color of injury in America's most popular sport', *Journal of Sport & Social Issues*, 41(4): 307–334.

Boxing England (2018) *England Boxing Rule Book*. London: England Boxing.

Brayton, S., Helstien, M., Ramsey, M., and Rickards, N. (2019) 'Exploring the missing link between the concussion "crisis" and labor politics in professional sports', *Communication and Sport*, 7(1): 110–131.

Bullingham, R., White, A., and Batten, J. (2017) 'Response to: "Don't let kids play football": a killer idea', *British Journal of Sports Medicine*, 51(20): 1450.

Cantu, R. and Hyman, M. (2012) *Concussions and our Kids*. Boston, MA: Mariner Books.

Carlisle, W. (2018) 'The AFL's concussion problem: is the league running interference on the damage concussion can cause?' www.themonthly.com.au/issue/2018/september/1535724000/wendy-carlisle/afl-s-concussion-problem

Carroll, L. and Rosner, D. (2011) *The Concussion Crisis: Anatomy of a Silent Epidemic*. New York: Simon and Schuster.

Cassilo, D. and Sanderson, J. (2018) '"I don't think it's worth the risk": media framing of the Chris Borland retirement in digital and print media', *Communication & Sport*, 6(1): 86–110.

Casson, I., Viano, D., Powell, J., and Pellman, E. (2010) 'Twelve years of National Football League concussion data', *Sport Health*, 2(6): 471–483.

Fainaru-Wada, M. and Fainaru, S. (2013) *League of Denial*. New York: Crown Business.

Furness, J. (2016) 'Reframing concussions, masculinity, and NFL mythology in League of Denial', *Popular Communication*, 14(1): 49–57.

Gilbert, F. and Partridge, B. (2012) 'The need to tackle concussion in Australian football codes', *Medical Journal of Australia*, 196(9): 561–563.

Goldberg, D. (2013) 'Mild traumatic brain injury, the National Football League, and the manufacture of doubt: an ethical, legal, and historical analysis', *Journal of Legal Medicine*, 34(2): 157–191.

Greenhow, A. (2018) *Why the Brain Matters: Regulating Concussion in Australian Sport*. Unpublished PhD thesis, Monash University, Melbourne Australia.

Greenhow, A. and East, J. (2015) 'Custodians of the game: ethical considerations for football governing bodies in regulating concussion management', *Neuroethics*, 8: 65–82.

Greenhow, A. and Gowthorp, L. (2017) 'Head injuries and concussion issues', in N. Shulenkorf and S. Frawley (eds.), *Critical Issues in Global Sports Management*, Abingdon, UK: Routledge, 93–112.

Grey-Thompson, Baroness T. (2017) *Duty of Care in Sport Review*. London: UK Govt. Department for Digital Culture, Media and Sport. www.gov.uk/government/publications/duty-of-care-in-sport-review

Gulland, A. (2018) 'Football headers and dementia: five minutes with Willie Stewart', *British Medical Journal*, 360: k190.

Hardes, J. (2017) 'Governing sporting brains: concussion, neuroscience, and the biopolitical regulation of sport', *Sport, Ethics & Philosophy*, 11(3): 281–293.

Hume, P., Theadom, A., Lewis, F., Quarrie, K., Brown, S., Hill, R., and Marshall, S. (2017) 'A comparison of cognitive function in former rugby union players compared with former non-contact-sport players and the impact of concussion history', *Sports Medicine*, 47: 1209–1220.

Kuhn, A., Yengo-Kahn, A., Kerr, Z., and Zuckerman, S. (2017) 'Sports concussion research, chronic traumatic encephalopathy and the media: repairing the disconnect,' *British Journal of Sports Medicine*, 51(24): 1732–1733.

Malcolm, D. (2017) *Sport, Medicine and Health: The Medicalization of Sport?* London: Routledge.

McGannon, K., Cunningham, S., and Schinke, R. (2013) 'Understanding concussion in socio-cultural context: a media analysis of a National Hockey League star's concussion', *Psychology of Sport and Exercise*, 14: 891–899.

Mrazik, M., Dennison, C., Brooks, B., Yeates, K.O., Babul, S., and Naidu, D. (2015) 'A qualitative review of sports concussion education: prime time for evidence-based knowledge translation', *British Journal of Sports Medicine*, 49: 1548–1553.

Partridge, B. (2014) 'Dazed and confused: sports medicine, conflicts of interest, and concussion management', *Bioethical Inquiry*, 11: 65–74.

Rugg, A. (2019) 'Civilizing the child: violence, masculinity, and race in media narratives of James Harrison', *Communication and Sport*, 7(1): 46–63.

Russell, K., Ellis, M., Bauman, S., and Tator, C. (2017) 'Legislation for youth sport concussion in Canada: review, conceptual framework, and recommendations', *Canadian Journal of Neurological Sciences*, 44(3): 225–234.

Sullivan, S., Schneiders, A., Cheang, C. et al. (2012) '"What's happening?" A content analysis of concussion-related traffic on Twitter', *British Journal of Sports Medicine*, 46: 258–263.

Ventresca, M. (2018) 'The curious case of CTE: mediating materialities of traumatic brain injury', *Communication and Sport*, doi:10.1177/2167479518761636

White, A., Batten, J., Kirkwood, G., Anderson, E., and Pollock, A. (2019) 'Pre-activity movement control exercise programme to prevent injuries in youth rugby: some concerns', *British Journal of Sports Medicine*, 53(9): 525–526.

Workewych, A., Muzzi, M., Jing, R., Zhang, S., Topolovec-Vranic, J., and Cusimano, M. (2017) 'Twitter and traumatic brain injury: a content and sentiment analysis of tweets pertaining to sport-related brain injury', *SAGE Open Medicine*, 5: 1–11.

4

CONCUSSION AND MEDICINE

'Funny, you're not the first person I've seen with this today,' the doctor said. The irritability and sleep disturbance Ash had described could be post-concussive syndrome, so she'd been advised to take things easy for a couple of weeks. This was the first time Ash had looked for help, but now she wished she hadn't bothered. 'Truth is, we don't really know too much about it,' the doctor concluded,

As we saw in Chapter 3, research has identified the failure of the media to accurately relay what is and is not known about concussion. Part of the explanation for this is the propensity for sensationalism in the reporting of scientific knowledge more broadly (Peters 2013), but it would be equally true to say that such sensationalist reporting is encouraged by the relatively high degrees of uncertainty that exist *within* the science of concussion. Thus, for commentators, politicians, and the public, gauging the accuracy and reliability of information is a challenge. While uncertainty may fuel the sense of crisis, equally it has been argued that uncertainty is a broader issue defining modern medicine (Fox 2000). Consequently, looking at the biomedical science of concussion in sport forwards our understanding of this crisis and tells us something about the relationship between medicine and society at large. But first, the key question we must ask is how significant have biomedical developments been, both in terms of enhancing our understanding of concussion and in terms of addressing the crisis?

While media representations of Bennet Omalu's 'discovery' of CTE shape popular cultural understandings of concussion science, Paul McCrory is perhaps a more significant individual. As editor of the *British Journal of Sports Medicine* from 2001–2008 he was prominent in criticizing existing research on concussion as, for instance, 'anecdotal . . . bizarre rather than reflecting established medical principles', a field plagued by 'neuromythology' derived from folk wisdom, methodologically flawed medical research, and media exposés of athletes' experiences of head trauma

(McCrory 2001: 82). The field was hampered, he said, by the lack of any 'existing animal or other experimental model that accurately reflects a sporting concussive injury' (McCrory et al. 2005: 197). Knowledge, rather, was based upon research examining head injuries sustained in either boxing or motor vehicle accidents, both of which were misleading because: 1) the frequency of repetitive head trauma in boxing was thought to pose 'unique risks'; and 2) collisions in sports such as rugby union involve much lower acceleration-deceleration forces than do motor vehicle accidents (although somewhat ironically subsequent research has highlighted both the relative frequency of head trauma in collision sports such as American football and the incidence of players experiencing forces which are comparable to those entailed in a car crash). McCrory (1999) further made the case that a proliferation of scales designed to assess the severity of head injuries (there were over 20 in 2000) simply created conflicting advice.

In subsequent years, biomedical concussion research would grow exponentially. Seminal in this field, however, are the consensus statements produced by the Concussion in Sport Group (CISG), which stem from a quadrennial meeting/ conference. The first publication of these was in 2002; the latest followed a meeting in Berlin in October 2016 and led to the publication of the fifth statement in early 2017. Indicative of the growing body of research, the latest consensus document claimed to have been developed following a review of 60,000 published studies. There are other consensus/position statements in existence. These have been published by bodies representing various medical specialisms, for example: the National Athletic Trainers' Association (Broglio et al. 2014), and the American Medical Society for Sports Medicine (AMSSM) (Harmon et al. 2013; Harmon et al. 2019); the Canadian Paediatric Society (Purcell 2012) and the American Academy of Pediatrics (Halstead et al. 2010); and the American Academy of Neurology (Giza et al. 2013) and the National Academy of Neuropsychology (Moser et al. 2007). An interorganizational statement of neuropsychological groups has also been published (Echemendia et al. 2012), as has a consensus statement of 'ringside physicians' (Neidecker et al. 2018). Each have their different merits, aims, and emphases. However, the CISG will be the focus here, partly because of its essentially global remit, but particularly because of its lineage. The production of a *series* of consensus statements enables us to both construct a relatively reliable biomedical knowledge base, but also to pursue the central aim of this chapter: namely, tracking how knowledge has developed over time to show how medical science both responds to and fuels sport's concussion crisis.

Aspects of this review of contemporary biomedical knowledge, we therefore look to establish: what we mean by concussion; what its signs and symptoms are; how patients can be assessed, managed, and rehabilitated; whether particular populations are at heightened risk; and how we might prevent concussions from occurring. In attempting to establish the boundaries of biomedical understanding in relation to concussion, we consider some of the key issues relating to SIS and CTE. In so doing we will also be able to identify: 1) how the knowledge base is expanding; 2) what is *not* known about concussion; and thus 3) how the complexities of understanding the human brain contribute to the concussion crisis. Before exploring the content of these statements, however, it is important to identify more clearly the human or social processes that lie behind their production.

Background and process

Tracking the sequence of CISG documents illustrates how the concussion statements have become more extensive, far-reaching, and politically self-conscious. For instance, in terms simply of length the publications have more than doubled, from four and a half pages in 2002 to more than nine in the latest iteration, peaking at 12 in 2013 (for simplicity's sake I will consistently use the date of publication rather than the meeting date). The reach of the consensus statements similarly appears to have grown. The 2002 statement was simultaneously published in three journals (*British Journal of Sports Medicine, Clinical Journal of Sports Medicine,* and *Physician and Sports Medicine*), which increased to nine in 2009. While the documents no longer make reference to parallel/duplicate publication, the digitalization of publishing and the opportunities of open access have effectively made these statements universally available. The authorship group has undergone a commensurate expansion from an original team of ten to 36, and the stated goals have changed from (simply) providing recommendations to improve athlete health and safety (2002) to guiding clinical practice and, more ambitiously, informing the agenda for future research (2017).

As the statements have become larger, drawn on a wider pool of expertise and enjoyed a broader impact, so claims for a position of authority have extended. The 2001 and 2005 documents are described as 'summary and agreement' statements, but the notion that these statements constituted a 'consensus' was introduced in 2009. At this point, there was an attempt to identify specific areas of unanimity. However, the word 'unanimous' only appeared five times in the 2009 document, and indeed twice it was noted that no unanimity was reached, leaving the level of agreement for most of the content undefined. In 2013 the CISG began to make more transparent the process behind the 'building' of consensus but noted that, 'while agreement exists pertaining to principal messages contained . . . the authors acknowledge that the science of concussion is evolving' (McCrory et al. 2013: 250). The 2017 statement is accompanied by a four-page summary of methodology (Meeuwisse et al. 2017), but how and where the agenda for these meetings is set remains unclear.

Even less clear is the evolving relationship between the statements' authors and external or vested interests in the wider sporting world. For instance, in 2002 it is clearly stated that the preceding symposium was organized by the IIHF, FIFA, and the International Olympic Committee (IOC). The composition of attendees reflected this, with six of the original ten listing an affiliation to one of these organizations. The statement further commends the three sports organizations for their 'enlightened' approach to concussion in sport (a phrase repeated in 2005, 2009, and 2013). The meeting for the 2005 statement was 'organised by the same group' (McCrory et al. 2005: 196), but in 2009 the first member affiliated to the

IRB attended, and the IRB is added to the list of governing bodies to be commended for their 'enlightened' outlook.[1] Yet concurrently there appears to have been an attempt to try to establish the independence of the CISG by distancing members of the group from the governing bodies. For instance, it is claimed that 'panellists . . . do not represent organisations per se but were selected for their expertise, experience and understanding of this field' (McCrory et al. 2009: i82). As the balance of vested interests continued to cause concern, the 2013 statement was accompanied by the publication of a ten-page supplementary file listing declared interests. While the 2017 statement reverts to the precedent set in 2002 through 2009 and simply states, 'None' under the authors' 'competing interests', this is contradicted by the 2017 methodological statement which describes the 'competing interests' of three people – including lead author Paul McCrory – who are named as authors in the broader consensus statement.

Thus, what at first appears to be an objective attempt to consolidate scientific knowledge must be seen as an inherently social and political process. More generally it has been argued that such consensus statements 'may be regarded as more a reflection of the desire of selected "experts" and scientists to impose their worldview on research and practice' (Bercovitz 2000), while specifically in relation to the CISG consensus statements, some have questioned 'whether the consensus is the outcome of predetermined selection rather than the conformity of scientific opinion' (McNamee et al. 2015: 194). Given a similar lack of transparency over the role of specific sports organizations, questions have also been asked about whether this 'could be seen as an attempt to steer the concussion agenda' and, ultimately, leads to the production of guidelines 'simply used to justify their own policies and practices' (McNamee et al. 2015: 194).

But these issues provide context to the documents rather than to dispute their underlying worth. The longevity of this group is indicative of a level of recognition within the biomedical field and is testament to the degree of authority with which such statements are received. They constitute what is, in many ways, the biomedical orthodoxy (see Chapter 9). An attempt to comprehensively cover the biomedical evidence from 'scratch' would, perhaps, be impossible for any individual and, certainly, beyond the remit of this book. Thus, despite the caveats raised, we can explore the CISG concussion statements to assess the development and current state of concussion science.

Defining concussion

At the outset, a need for both a more applicable and more widely accepted definition of concussion was identified. Existing models, such as that endorsed by the American Medical Association and the International Neurotraumatology Association, were thought to fail to sufficiently capture the kinds of concussion seen in sport, particularly in terms of the range of symptoms manifest and their potential to occur following relatively minor impacts (Aubrey et al. 2002). Specifically, since the 1966 Congress of Neurological Surgeons consensus definition, the main emphasis had been placed on brain stem dysfunction and loss of consciousness (Greenhow 2018). Thus, in 2002 a new definitional statement was produced and, despite some slight amendments to the wording since, the essence of that text has remained largely unchanged. The CISG's current definition is provided as follows, with bold text used to signify the major changes added since the first iteration:

> Sport related concussion [SRC] is a traumatic brain injury induced by bio-mechanical forces. Several common features that may be utilised in clinically defining the nature of a concussive head injury include:
>
> - SRC may be caused either by a direct blow to the head, face, neck or elsewhere on the body with an impulsive force transmitted to the head.
> - SRC typically results in the rapid onset of short-lived impairment of neurological function that resolves spontaneously. **However, in some cases, signs and symptoms evolve over a number of minutes to hours**.
> - SRC may result in neuropathological changes, but the acute clinical signs and symptoms largely reflect a functional disturbance rather than a structural injury and, as such, no abnormality is seen on standard structural neuroimaging studies.
> - SRC results in a range of clinical signs and symptoms that may or may not involve loss of consciousness. Resolution of the clinical and cognitive features typically follows a sequential course. **However, in some cases symptoms may be prolonged**.
>
> **The clinical signs and symptoms cannot be explained by drug, alcohol, or medication use, other injuries (such as cervical injuries, peripheral vestibular dysfunction, etc) or other comorbidities (e.g., psychological factors or coexisting medical conditions)**.
>
> *(McCrory et al. 2017: 2)*

Thus the key points of change have been to: 1) add clauses related to the evolution of concussion in terms of both the development and duration of symptoms over time; and 2) recognize that symptoms may be attributable to other causes which therefore need to be ruled-out before concussion is diagnosed.

But while the CISG's definition has been relatively stable, dissatisfaction continues to be expressed over the use of terminology. Despite divisions between those countries for whom English is a primary language, and continental Europe where *commotion cerebri* is a widely used term (McCrory et al. 2013), the debate about the relationship between the terms concussion and mTBI has frequently been revisited. In this regard, it is particularly notable that the CISG changed its terminology in the latest document. The first reference to 'sport-related concussion' (SRC) rather than simply concussion was introduced in 2017, perhaps signalling a move to formalize this as an essentially independent condition. Fuelling this movement has been the development of an awareness/belief that concussion has broader and more varied manifestations than previously thought. This in turn has been accompanied by an increasingly explicit identification of how complicated sport-related concussions are, such that in 2013 it was stated that concussion is 'among the most complex injuries in sports medicine to diagnose, assess and manage' (McCrory et al. 2013: 7). The longstanding and relatively stable nature of the agreement upon a definition provides evidence of continuity of understanding, but the view that sport-specific conditions are distinct from the head trauma experienced in other spheres of social life seems to have been one of the more significant developments in recent years. This development should be seen in the context of what appears to be increasingly acrimonious relations between members of the 'sports medicine' and those working in neuroscience (Sharp and Jenkins 2015). UK neurologist Willie Stewart, for instance, is reported to have said of the CISG consensus document, 'This is not science, this isn't experts, this isn't medicine, this is sport [that] has written the document' (Carlisle 2018).

The signs and symptoms of concussion

A second founding principle has been for these statements to provide guidance on the signs and symptoms of 'acute concussion'. The earliest statement identified a range of cognitive features, typical symptoms, and physical signs (see Table 4.1). However, by 2009 these were expanded to five categories: symptoms (somatic and emotional); physical signs; behavioural changes; cognitive impairment; and sleep disturbance. Most recently (2017) a sixth category – balance impairment – was included, although essentially this is a recategorization rather than expansion of signs and symptoms. Evidence of any one of these can be taken to be indicative of the *possibility* of concussion. Implicitly, therefore, there is relatively little emphasis on the *chronic* signs and symptoms of concussion.

TABLE 4.1 The signs and symptoms of concussion (Aubrey et al. 2002)

Domain	Manifestation
Cognitive features	unaware of period, opposition, or score of game; confusion; amnesia; loss of consciousness; unaware of time, date, place
Typical symptoms	headache, dizziness, nausea, unsteadiness/loss of balance, feeling 'dinged' or stunned or 'dazed', 'having my bell rung', seeing stars of flashing lights, ringing in the ears, double vision, others (including sleepiness, sleep disturbance, feeling of slowness and fatigue)
Physical signs	loss of consciousness/impaired conscious state, poor coordination or balance, concussive convulsion/impact seizure, gait unsteadiness/loss of balance, slow to answer questions or follow directions, easily distracted/poor concentration, display of inappropriate emotions, nausea/vomiting, vacant stare/glassy eyed, slurred speech, personality changes, inappropriate playing behaviour, appreciably decreased playing ability

But despite considerable continuity in how we recognize the potential existence of concussion, the symptoms remain diffuse and heterogeneous and there continues to be no particular symptom or combination of symptoms which is either necessary or sufficient to make a definitive diagnosis. Confounding factors include the evidence that people who experience one concussion seem to be more likely to report subsequent occurrences, or that over time more pronounced symptoms seem to stem from more minor trauma. The CISG statements remain notably silent on the issue of SIS even though the condition was first discussed by Schneider (1973) 45 years ago, and high profile incidents (e.g. Ben Robinson discussed in Chapter 2) suggest that it is children who are predominantly affected by this 'condition' (Gilbert and Partridge 2012). Both in relation to the greater frequency and severity of subsequent or multiple concussions, a major issue appears to be an inability to identify specifically why these patterns might be observed. Potentially therefore the data may be influenced by subjective or self-report bias.

Perhaps because of this, an ongoing preoccupation of these statements has been the desire to give guidance on which signs/symptoms provide the best indication of injury severity. For instance, the 2001 statement both spoke of the 'renewed interest' in the significance of amnesia (relative to loss of consciousness) and explored the idea that different concussion subtypes might exist. A distinction between simple and complex concussions was introduced in 2005 but was withdrawn from 2009 onwards. Scepticism over the use of grading scales for concussion in sport has, however, been consistent. The popularity of these scales was no doubt partly inspired by the broader brain injury research where such classificatory systems are deemed useful (e.g. the Glasgow Coma Scale); however, no single scale has been explicitly accepted for assessing SRC since 2005. Their rejection may have been an attempt to move past an area evidently lacking in consensus and away from the conventions practised in many sports, whereby coaches and players see loss of consciousness as the primary if not the sole defining symptom of concussion (see Chapter 6). But equally they also substantiate the claim for the distinctiveness of *sport-related* concussion as a condition. In place of such scales was guidance that 'the majority (80–90 per cent) of concussions resolve in a short (7–10 day) period, although the recovery time frame may be longer in children and adolescents' (McCrory et al. 2009: i77). The most recent guidance refers only to 'normal clinical recovery' periods, but these have now been extended to 10–14 days for adults, and in excess of 4 weeks for children. It is not clearly stated but one reading of this is that those who experience symptoms for less than 7–10 days (i.e. the 'normal clinical recovery' period) may *not* be defined as having sustained a concussion injury.

A final feature of the signs and symptoms which has consistently been addressed is the absence of reliable diagnostic tools/techniques. Since 2002 there has been support for the value of neuropsychological assessment of concussion, but even in the most recent statement this is not deemed sufficiently reliable to: 1) advocate any specific method; or 2) recommend that baseline testing of athletes be mandatory. In 2004 a Sport Concussion Assessment Tool (SCAT) was introduced that sought to consolidate existing tools. It included assessment of observable signs (consciousness, seizures, and balance), memory tests, patients' score of symptoms, cognitive assessment (through word recall and sequence reversal), and neurologic screening (speech, eye movement, gait, and pronator or muscle extension). The two-page test has expanded to eight pages in the most recent version (SCAT5; see also the section on special populations).[2] In 2009 objective balance assessment was cited as an effective diagnostic tool – on a par with neuropsychological assessment – but the view remained that the use of neuroimaging 'contributes little to concussion evaluation' (McCrory et al. 2009: i77), and that genetic testing and other experimental methods of assessment (e.g. different electrophysiological techniques and biomarkers) could not (yet) be justified. By 2017 we see reports of 'major progress in clinical methods for evaluation', but recognition that 'advanced neuroimaging, fluid biomarkers and genetic testing . . . require further validation to determine their ultimate clinical utility in evaluation of SRC' (McCrory et al. 2017: 4–5). As a consequence of the continued absence of a technological solution for the diagnosis of concussion, the recommendation continues as originally stated; the management of concussion should 'remain largely in the realm of clinical judgement on an individual basis' (Aubrey et al. 2002: 9).

Management and rehabilitation from concussion

As with diagnosis, the central strategy for the management of concussion has remained largely static since 2002, with the recommendation that any player showing any of the signs or symptoms of concussion should be immediately removed from play. Caution is urged; 'When in doubt, sit them out' (Aubrey et al. 2002: 8). The athlete, subsequently, should not be allowed to return to the field of play, should not be left alone (for approximately 48 hours), and should be regularly monitored and medically supervised through a stepwise RTP process. Indeed, not only has this not altered since 2002, it has not significantly changed for 70 years, for as we saw in Chapter 2, the notion that the concussed boxer should rest and abstain from sporting activity has been widely accepted since around 1945. Physical rest remained the sole recommendation for rehabilitation until 2005 when it was supplemented with 'cognitive rest' (see the section on special populations for further discussion).

Those injury management protocols signal how little the sports medicine doctor can offer the concussed athlete in terms of relieving or resolving their condition and how little new evidence for effective treatment has emerged. Indeed, in 2013 it was conceded that the evidence for recommending rest was 'sparse', and even now it is stated that while rest may ease discomfort and promote faster recovery, 'there is currently insufficient evidence that prescribing complete rest achieves these objectives' (McCrory et al. 2017: 5). We might further question whether the concept of cognitive rest is at all meaningful; can we stop thinking (Craton and Leslie 2014)? What we *have* seen, however, is the RTP protocol become more formalized and increasingly detailed, with the concussed athlete – once initial symptoms have resolved – guided through a six-stage graduated RTP, progressively building up aerobic activity and physical contact. Caveats to this standardization have been proposed – the idea expressed in 2005 that under the guidance of an experienced doctor RTP was often quicker, and the 2009 citation of NFL data which suggested that some players could RTP on the same day with no ill-effects – but notably no such sub-clauses remain. While there has been a drift towards more elongated rehabilitation periods, the emotional appeal of a RTP protocol that coincides with the weekly basis of many sporting competitions continues to be strong. There is scope for concussed athletes to return to competition in seven days even though, within the terms set by the CISG, this amounts to between 50 per cent and 70 per cent of the currently defined 'normal recovery period'. Indeed it has recently been claimed that 80 per cent of concussed players in the AFL are declared fit to play the following week and thus miss no competitive matches (Carlisle 2018).

Finally, in relation to rehabilitation, there is a distinct absence of effective interventions. There is an increasingly explicit consideration of how post-concussive depression can be managed, and there is some 'preliminary evidence' supporting the use of physical and cognitive behavioural therapies (including undertaking light exercise), but it remains the case that 'there is limited evidence supporting the use of pharmacotherarpy' and indeed a concern that medication may only mask symptoms and so potentially do more harm than good (McCrory et al. 2017: 5). The 2013 document is interesting in acknowledging that a range of commercially available technological devices have become available, but equally for expressing caution as 'only limited evidence exists for their role in this setting and none have been validated as diagnostic' (McCrory et al. 2013: 257).

Special populations

In one of the few distinct departures from the original document, the 2005 statement began the process of differentiating between the effects of concussion on different populations. In the language of biomedicine 'special populations' can be any group requiring additional or targeted investigation but in relation to concussion, as we saw briefly in Chapters 2 and 3, most specialist concern has been directed towards the protection of youth athletes. First, however, we explore concerns about gender differences and the impact of concussion on occupationally specific groups.

Gender received its first mention in the 2009 CISG statements. However, because it has always been cited as a possible 'modifying factor' rather than a special population consideration, the primary hypothesis appears to be that the differences are social rather than biological, or at least potentially open to intervention. In both 2009 and 2013 it is stated that 'although it was accepted that gender may be a risk factor for injury and/or influence injury severity' (McCrory et al. 2013: 253), there was no unanimity over the relationship between gender and concussion. While in 2009 gender was identified as a key future research area, by 2017 mention is reduced simply to noting that girls appear to have greater risk than boys of suffering *persistent* symptoms (thus conflating the influence of gender with age). Consequently the medical evidence for treating males and females differently remains limited and unclear.

Conversely discussion of CTE in the section on special populations (which appears from 2009) implicitly signals an understanding that the condition should not be a broader public health concern, but an occupationally specific outcome. The framing of CTE in this way is indicative of the particularly CTE-sceptic character of the CISG statements (McNamee et al. 2015. See Chapter 5, this volume, for a discussion of the ethical issues in relation to this). While the cited literature has expanded over time, the statements continue to conclude that the evidence is not, '*at this stage*', sufficiently compelling and that 'a cause and effect relationship has not *as yet* been demonstrated between CTE and concussions or exposure to contact sports' (McCrory et al. 2009: i80, emphasis added). The way the 2009 document provided five supporting references regarding 'anecdotal' case reports, but none to the 'epidemiological studies . . . [which] suggested an association between repeated sports concussions during a career and late life cognitive impairment' provides another illustration of this point (McCrory et al. 2009: i80), for it is unconventional for medical consensus statements to give such precedence to anecdotal evidence over published epidemiological studies. While the 2017 statement is accompanied by a systematic review incorporating 47 studies, it still concluded that 'multiple concussions appear to be a risk factor for cognitive impairment and mental health problems in *some* individuals' and called for more research in this area (Manley et al. 2017: 1, emphasis added). These concerns, it argued, should be balanced against the expressed need to address 'fears of parents/ athletes [derived] from media pressure' (McCrory et al. 2013: 254). The consensus position continues to be that, 'the notion that repeated concussion or sub-concussive impacts cause CTE remains unknown' (Manley et al. 2017: 7).[3]

In contrast, concerns over 'paediatric concussive injury' are prominent. This section was introduced in 2005 and initially it was simply stated that the prior guidance designed for adult males was relevant to the management of children (defined as 5–18 years old). It was in this context that the idea of cognitive rest as recuperative was first introduced. Specifically, the text referred to relief from academic work, with examples of daily living such as sending text messages and playing video games introduced in 2009. The 2005 statement noted that neuropsychological testing was *less reliable* for children due to the relatively significant 'cognitive maturation' that occurs during these ages. Whilst stressing the inherent uncertainty via calls for research to clarify the value of cognitive assessment tools and the differences between adult and child responses to concussion, it has been repeatedly recommended that more conservative protocols (including longer 'normal' recovery periods and extended RTP) should be applied to children.

By 2009 the third consensus statement prioritized 'paediatric concussions' as one of five 'focus questions'. It provided some support for more conservative approaches due to 'the different physiological response and longer recovery after concussion and specific risks (e.g. diffuse cerebral swelling) related to head impact during childhood and adolescence' (McCrory et al. 2009: i80), but also warned of the greater complexity generated by learning and hyperactivity disorders among children, and identified the need for parent and/or teacher input in clinical evaluation. The document further claimed that 'head injury rates are often higher' amongst children and adolescents than adult athletes (McCrory et al. 2009: i81) and, by 2013, this precipitated the introduction of a child SCAT and a recommendation for the deployment of specialist neuropsychologists to assess paediatric cases. But crucially what constitutes a 'child' has continued to be redefined without explanation. The 2009 document revised the scope of existing recommendations (now deemed applicable down to the age of 10 rather than 5), but in 2012 the key distinction is drawn at 13 years of age. Further nuance appears in 2017 distinguishing between children (5–12 years of age) and adolescents (13–18 years of age). Yet as noted previously, the documents make no reference to any qualitatively distinct manifestation of concussion in youth (e.g. in relation to SIS) suggesting this remains contested.

The increasing tenor of conservatism when dealing with children therefore seems to be driven by paternalistic concerns rather than biomedical advancement. For instance, the 2013 document contained certain statements – 'children should not be returned to sport until clinically completely symptom-free'; 'it is not appropriate for a child or adolescent athlete with concussion to RTP on the same day as injury' (McCrory et al. 2013: 254) – which are essentially redundant given that this advice applies to all athletes, regardless of age. The 2017 statement seemed to endorse legislative changes seen in the US (see Chapter 3), encouraging schools to have sport-related concussion policies and drafting a 'return to school' strategy which prioritizes return to learning over any RTP concerns. It cites histories of mental health and migraines as particularly significant for children, adolescents, and 'young adults' (an additional but undefined term, see McCrory et al. 2017: 6). But most significantly it signals that the distinctions drawn are essentially precautionary rather than evidence-based. It notes that the 'paucity of studies that are specific to children, especially younger children, needs to be addressed as a priority', that 'the literature does not adequately address' the different management of children and adults with concussion, and that 'no studies have addressed whether sport-related concussion signs and symptoms differ from adults' (McCrory et al. 2017: 7). This ethically inspired conservatism has social roots that are discussed further in Chapter 8.

Prevention

In light of the previous discussion, and given the continued recognition that 'the ability to treat or reduce the effects of concussive injury after the event is minimal' (McCrory et al. 2005: 202), the role of prevention has gradually become more prominent. Based on an initial concern that 'the brain is not an organ that can be conditioned to withstand injury' and the view that 'there is little scientific evidence' that neck muscle conditioning could reduce injuries (Aubrey et al. 2002: 9), successive statements have looked at the role of protective equipment, rule changes/enforcement and cultural change, and education or knowledge transfer.

The efficacy of protective equipment is perhaps one of the most consistently addressed issues in these documents. It has generally been found that both mouthguards and helmets offer protection from other injuries, but not concussion. The sports cited in the documents change over time (initially baseball, grid iron and ice hockey were cited but these sports were replaced by cycling, equestrianism, and alpine and motor sports in 2009, signalling again the spill-over characteristics of a cultural crisis). Mention of the NFL is a conspicuous absence. But there also appears to be an underlying scepticism about protective equipment as a solution, for in 2009 the CISG argued that current biomechanical research had shown that while such equipment could reduce impacts, this had not been translated into consistently reduced rates of concussion. Indeed, since 2005 statements have continued to raise the issue of 'risk compensation', or the idea that the use of protective equipment results in behavioural changes leading, paradoxically, to increased injury rates. As such, these statements seem to support those who advocate more limited changes to the way sports are played.

These technological 'failures' have meant that the rule changes and stricter rule enforcement described in Chapter 3 provide 'a key role in reducing and preventing concussions' (Aubrey et al. 2002: 4). The prohibition of head-checking in ice hockey was initially cited as a good example (McCrory et al. 2005), as was restricting heading contests in soccer, through which contact between players' arms and heads were believed to account for 50 per cent of all concussions in the game (note the concern here is *not* about heading the ball per se, but about the contact incurred in the process of heading. The statements make no reference to soccer, heading, and longer-term neurocognitive decline). Emphasis has, however, shifted from the centrality of the referee in ensuring rule adherence to rule changes enabling medical assessment, 'without compromising the athlete's welfare, affecting the flow of the game or unduly penalising the player's team' (McCrory et al. 2009: i81). The CISG, moreover, pronounces that while it is the duty of sports organizations to ensure fair and respectful play between opponents as a way of limiting injuries, the 'essence' of these activities (as they see it), should not be changed: 'the competitive/aggressive nature of sport which makes it fun to play and watch should not be discouraged' (McCrory et al. 2009. Note that the changed aims of the CISG statements mean that such recommendations fall outside the scope of the 2017 version and, consequently, such arguments have been replaced with recommendations for future research).

The desire to shape the ethos by which sports are played leads to consideration of what was initially termed education and has subsequently been described as knowledge transfer (KT). Ensuring that players behave ethically forms one component of this KT, but it is also perceived that athletes should be (better) informed about how to detect concussion and how to RTP safely. While discussed in more detail in Chapter 7, two points need to be made here. First, in making these pronouncements the CISG appears to go beyond its medical expertise and into ethical

What we do see fairly consistently in the epidemiological data is a ranking of incidence across sports. Generally speaking, lower rates appear in sports such as volleyball, cheerleading, and baseball, and the highest rates relate to collision sports such as American football, rugby, and hockey (Pfister et al. 2016). Fighting sports such as boxing and taekwondo provide indicative evidence of even higher rates, but studies are too small or too few in number for meaningful conclusions to be drawn. While cross-cultural variability in popularity of particular sports, and differing gender dynamics, also inhibits comparison, especially soccer, where European participation is disproportionately male, yet female in North America, females are believed to report more concussions than males (Daneshvar et al. 2011), and youths are thought to report more concussions than adults (Pfister et al. 2016). Most unequivocal, though, is the growth in reported concussion rates over time. Hospitalizations for concussion in Victoria, Australia, increased by 60.5 per cent between 2002–2003 and 2010–2011 (Finch and Clapperton 2013). NCAA data show a doubling of concussion incidence over 15 years (1988–1989 to 2003–2004) (Daneshvar et al. 2011). Reported concussions rose fivefold at the five at FIFA World Cups held between 1998 and 2014 (Junge and Dvorak 2015).

It is difficult to assess the degree to which these data trends *explain* the major concerns of the concussion crisis in sport, and to what extent they *mirror* them. However, there are clear parallels between these data sets and the headline issues of this crisis – the incidence of concussion appears to be rising, making concussion a concern for a broader and broader range of activities, and the greatest concerns are expressed in relation to the sports participation of children and girls in particular. But as seen elsewhere in this chapter, the gaps in this body of scientific knowledge lead these concerns to spring from a mixture of fact and paternalistic speculation. Consequently, the scope that exists for different interpretations of epidemiological data epitomizes how medical research effectively fuels the notion of crisis in relation to concussion in sport.

The link between epidemiology and broader cultural concerns is problematic because the limitations of such quantification are fundamental to the discipline. Marshall and Spencer's (2001) review of ten studies of concussion in rugby union found that while estimates of all injuries varied by a factor of about ten, estimates of concussion injuries varied by a factor close to 100. They attributed such differences to the definition of injury and the method of injury data collection used in these respective surveys. But what they did *not* note, and what was equally evident, was the cross-cultural variation in estimates of incidence. Their conclusion that there must be a 'hidden epidemic' of concussion in rugby (see Chapter 1 for reflections on the use of that term) was based on a comparison of their US data against that generated by studies by South African, Australian, British and New Zealand researchers. Such cross-cultural variation in incidence rates has been replicated in other studies, for instance, comparisons of concussion rates in football across different European leagues (Walden et al. 2013).

As we established in Chapter 3, sport's concussion crisis manifests itself differently in different cultural contexts. Given such diversity it is important to reflect on the nature of the 'truth' we are seeking to clarify. The inescapable conclusion from epidemiological studies (of concussion) is that they seek to objectively quantify what is a qualitative or subjective social experience. Given that the biomedical experts assembled to inform the CISG consensus statements identify concussion as amongst the most complex conditions to diagnose (hence the recommended deferral to individual clinical judgement), what hope is there of assembling meaningful prevalence data? After all, estimates of prevalence rely on surveys of often retrospective, self-report of 'patient' symptoms and/or on multiple and varied clinical opinions. In Chapter 6 we explore what behavioural science has revealed about the lived experience of concussion, including reflections on clinicians' attempts at diagnosis. Our more immediate task is to look at the ethical issues evoked by the concussions crisis, identifying how these have come to inform both the broader social response to concussion and, as we have seen here, the production of medical knowledge.

Notes

1 Confusingly the 2013 document identifies 2005 as the beginning of the rugby authorities' involvement in these talks, but personnel-wise there is no evidence to support this claim.
2 The renumbering of the SCAT tests aligns with the conference at which it was revised rather than the actual version of the test. Similarly, the first Concussion Recognition Test – CRT3 – was introduced in 2013. The CRT was designed for use by those without prior medical training.
3 It is important to reiterate the degree of uncertainty relating to CTE here. A recent statement by a group of leading neuropathologists in the UK was at pains to stress that: 1) CTE is not yet fully defined; 2) understanding of the pathology is incomplete; and 3) diagnostic criteria are preliminary only, so current statements related to identification of CTE merely represent opinions (as another pathologist might reach a different conclusion). Conversely, they note, 'Too often an inaccurate impression is portrayed that CTE is clinically defined, its prevalence is high, and pathology evaluation is a simple positive or negative decision' (Stewart et al. 2019: 232)

References

Aubrey, M., Cantu, R., Dvorak, J., et al. (2002) 'Summary and agreement statement of the first international conference on concussion in sport, Vienna 2001', *British Journal of Sports Medicine*, 36: 6–10.
Bercovitz, K. (2000) 'A critical analysis of Canada's "Active Living": science or politics?', *Critical Public Health*, 10(1): 19–39.
Broglio, S., Cantu, R., Gioia, G., Guskiewicz, K., Palm, M., and McLeod, T. (2014) 'National Athletic Trainers' Association position statement: management of concussion in sport', *Journal of Athletic Training*, 49(2): 245–265.
Carlisle, W. (2018) 'The AFL's concussion problem: Is the league running interference on the damage concussion can cause?' www.themonthly.com.au/issue/2018/september/1535724000/wendy-carlisle/afl-s-concussion-problem
Craton, N. and Leslie, O. (2014) 'Time to re-think the Zurich guidelines? A critique on the consensus statement on concussion in sport, held in Zurich, November 2012', *Clinical Journal of Sports Medicine*, 24(2): 93–95.

Daneshvar, D., Nowinski, C., McKee, A., and Cantu, R. (2011) 'The epidemiology of sport-related concussion', *Clinical Sports Medicine*, 30(1): 1–17.

Echemendia, R., Iverson, G.McCrea, M. et al. (2012) 'Role of neuropsychologists in the evaluation and management of sport-related concussion: an inter-organization position statement', *Archives of Clinical Neuropsychology*, 27: 119–122.

Finch, C. and Clapperton, A. (2013) 'Increasing incidence of hospitalization for sport-related concussion in Victoria, Australia', *Medical Journal of Australia*, 198(8): 1–4.

Fox, R.C. (2000) 'Medical uncertainty revisited', in G.L. Albrecht, R. Fitzpatrick, and S.C. Scrimshaw (eds.), *The Handbook of Social Studies in Health and Medicine*. London: SAGE, 409–425.

Gilbert, F. and Partridge, B. (2012) 'The need to tackle concussion in Australian football codes', *Medical Journal of Australia*, 196(9): 561–563.

Giza, C., Kurcher, J., Ashwal, S. et al. (2013) 'Summary of evidence-based guideline update: evaluation and management of concussion in sports', *Neurology*, 80: 2250–2257.

Greenhow, A. (2018) *Why the Brain Matters: Regulating Concussion in Australian Sport.* Unpublished PhD thesis, Monash University, Melbourne Australia.

Halstead, M., Walter, K., and The Council on Sports Medicine and Fitness (2010) 'Sport-related concussion in children and adolescents', *Pediatrics*, 126: 597–615.

Harmon, K., Clugston, J., Dec, K. et al. (2019) 'American Medical Society for Sports Medicine position statement: concussion in sport', *British Journal of Sports Medicine*, 53: 213–225.

Harmon, K., Drezner, J., Gammons, M., Guskiewicz, K., Halstead, M., Herring, S., Kutcher, J., Pana, A., Putukian, M., and Roberts, W. (2013) 'American Medical Society for Sports Medicine position statement: concussion in sport', *British Journal of Sports Medicine*, 47: 15–26.

Junge, A. and Dvorak, J. (2015) 'Football injuries during the 2014 FIFA World Cup', *British Journal of Sports Medicine*, 49: 599–602.

Manley, G., Gardner, A., Schneider, K. et al. (2017) 'A systematic review of potential long-term effects of sport-related concussion', *British Journal of Sports Medicine*, 51: 969–977.

Marshall, S. and Spencer, R. (2001) 'Concussion in rugby: the hidden epidemic', *Journal of Athletic Training*, 36(3): 334–338.

McCrory, P. (1999) 'You can run but you can't hide: the role of concussion severity scales in sport', *British Journal of Sports Medicine*, 33: 297–298.

McCrory, P. (2001) 'When to retire after concussion?', *British Journal of Sports Medicine*, 35: 81–82.

McCrory, P., Johnston, K., Meeuwisse, W. et al. (2005) 'Summary and agreement statement of the 2nd international conference on concussion in sport, Prague 2004', *British Journal of Sports Medicine*, 39: 196–204.

McCrory, P., Meeuwisse, W., Aubrey, M. et al. (2013) 'Consensus statement on concussion in sport: the 4th international conference on concussion in sport held in Zurich, November 2012', *British Journal of Sports Medicine*, 47: 250–258.

McCrory, P., Meeuwisse, W., Dvorak, J. et al. (2017) 'Consensus statement on concussion in sport: the 5th international conference on concussion in sport held in Berlin, October 2016', *British Journal of Sports Medicine*, 51: 838–847.

McCrory, P., Meeuwisse, W., Johnston, K. et al. (2009) 'Consensus statement on concussion in sport: the 3rd international conference on concussion in sport held in Zurich, November 2008', *British Journal of Sports Medicine*, 43(Suppl 1): i76–i80.

McNamee, M., Partridge, B., and Anderson, L. (2015) 'Concussion in sport: conceptual and ethical issues', *Kinesiology Review*, 4: 190–202.

Meeuwisse, W., Schneider, K., Dvorka, J., Omu, O., Finch, C., Hayden, K., and McCrory, P. (2017) 'The Berlin process: a summary of methodology for the 5th international consensus conference on concussion in sport', *British Journal of Sports Medicine*, 51: 873–876.

Moser, R., Iverson, G., Echmendia, R, et al. (2007) 'Neuropsychological evaluation in the diagnosis and management of sports-related concussion', *Archives of Clinical Neuropsychology*, 22: 909–916.

Neidecker, J., Sethi, N., TaylorR. et al. (2018) 'Concussion management in combat sports: consensus statement from the Association of Ringside Physicians', *British Journal of Sports Medicine*, Online First: 26 July 2018. doi:10.1136/bjsports-2017–098799

Peters, H. (2013) 'Gap between science and media revisited: scientists as public communicators', *Proceedings of the National Academy of Sciences of the United States of America*, 110(3): 14102–14109.

Pfister, T., Pfister, K., Hagel, B., Ghali, W., and Ronksley, P. (2016) 'The incidence of concussion in youth sports: a systematic review and meta-analysis', *British Journal of Sports Medicine*, 50: 292–297.

Purcell, L. (2012) 'Evaluation and management of children and adolescents with sport-related concussion', *Paediatric Child Health*, 17(1): 31–32.

Schneider, R.C. (1973) *Head and Neck Injuries in Football: Mechanisms, Treatment, and Prevention*. Baltimore, MD: Williams & Wilkins.

Sharp, D. and Jenkins, P. (2015) 'Concussion is confusing us all', *Practical Neurology*, 15: 172–186.

Stewart, W., Allinson, K., Al-Sarraj, S. et al. (2019) 'Primum non nocere: a call for balance when reporting CTE', *Lancet Neurology*, 18: 231–232.

Walden, M., Hagglund, M., Orchard, J., Kristenson, K., and Ekstrand, J. (2013) 'Regional differences in injury incidence in European professional football', *Scandinavian Journal of Medicine & Science in Sports*, 23: 424–430.

5

CONCUSSION AND ETHICS

Ash had played big games with injuries before. She'd just be careful. But Ash's mum explained that brains were different, that you just never knew when the damage would appear. That was why they had put all those rules in place. 'I know you're not a kid, but you're my daughter. I can't let you play'.

Contributing to the reasons why concussion, rather than sports injury in general, has generated a cultural crisis is the range and complexity of the ethical issues involved. To fully understand sport's concussion crisis, we therefore need to review some of the detail of these debates in order to become more sensitive to the ethical considerations involved. The aim of this chapter is *not* to provide resolutions to the ethical dilemmas, but to develop an understanding of the underpinning issues which, in turn, have governance and regulatory implications.

To that end, the chapter is divided into three parts which explore ethical considerations that arise from the science, regulation, and the day-to-day medical practice related to concussion injuries. While separated here for ease of understanding there is, in reality, considerable overlap between these areas. As we saw in Chapter 4, scientific knowledge informs regulation which filters down to structure medical practice. Additionally, it should be noted that this is not a simple cause and effect model, where ethical issues 'create' a crisis or direct medical science and practice. Rather the perception of crisis, as well as greater regulation and more proactive governance, may all evoke new ethical considerations. Why does SRC present such difficult problems?

Science

All branches of biomedical research entail their own distinct ethical considerations. Genetics, for instance, poses ethical questions about the 'ownership' of essentially intergenerational information (in what circumstances do children have a right to their parents' medical records?). Neuroscience is similarly distinct, but mainly because of the ethical issues that relate to the specific organ in question. Neuroethics has thus developed as a field devoted to interrogating the potential consequences of medical practice and research on the brain (Fry and MacNamee 2017). In this section we explore ethical issues which largely stem from our inability to precisely identify concussion (and related conditions) and the attempts of certain actors to create a scientific orthodoxy which ameliorates such uncertainty (specifically through the production of Concussion in Sport Group consensus statements). However, our discussion of the ethics of concussion science must start with a more fundamental question: how, and in what ways, do we understand the brain to be distinct from other bodily organs?

Neuroscience and concussion

The distinctiveness of the brain as a human organ can be seen in what have been called 'paradoxical cognitive phenomena' (Fry 2017: 301). These might include cases where cognitive deficits seem to accompany neurological benefits (as portrayed in some accounts that link bipolar disorders to heightened creativity) or alleviation of a cognitive deficit following a second brain lesion ('double hit recovery'). But perhaps more socially pervasive is the distinctiveness encapsulated in Descartes' mind-body dualism. Since the seventeenth century, beliefs that the mind is both separate from and different to the body (the mind being part of the brain) have been dominant in Western thought. Thus, while the body is conceived of as a physical and somewhat 'mechanical' entity, the mind is *more* than this, housing consciousness, self-awareness, identity. Indeed, more or less everything which makes us human and distinguishes us from other living beings is attributed to the mind/brain. The brain is widely seen as a sacrosanct organ because it is perceived to hold the 'essence' of the person in much the same way that the heart once was (Greenhow and Gowthorp 2017; Johnson Thornton 2011).

This distinctiveness translates into a parallel sense in which brain injuries 'don't fit preconceived ideas of what injury "looks" like' (Fry 2017: 297). There are three main dimensions to this: transparency, flexibility, and immediacy. Some injuries are visible to the human eye or detectable through physical examination. Others may require imaging techniques such as X-rays or MRI scans to render them understandable. But, as noted in Chapter 4, despite considerable endeavours, brain injuries, and in particular SRCs, are frequently beyond definitive identification. It is for this reason that evidence from the post-mortem autopsies of former NFL athletes has assumed such significance; it appears more definitive. But because our knowledge of the brain is at its most complete only after a person dies, there are inevitable ethical dilemmas about the 'right' point in time at which medical or social interventions should occur.

Second, contemporary neuroscience emphasizes the plasticity of the brain (Johnson Thornton 2011). The responsiveness of the brain to external stimuli (from reading to banging one's head) raises questions about which brain changes should be regarded as pathological and which are merely within the 'normal' range of brain adaptation. As Fry (2017: 297) poses, 'does brain injury require a noticeable cognitive deficit, emotional disturbance (conscious or otherwise) or other functional impairment?' Currently we do not know, but we have nevertheless seen significant changes (e.g. the ban on types of tackling described in Chapter 3) that are based on the answer being 'no'. Alternatively, to what extent does the brain have the capacity to 'rewire' and therefore compensate for its own injuries? Can it, in certain circumstances, heal itself? Finally, can we assume that every psychological condition has an underlying brain pathology (and it is just that we do not have the technical capability to detect it)? Put another way, are we right to assume a link between the manifestation of depression and patterns of tau proteins in the brain that are used in the diagnosis of Chronic Traumatic Encephalopathy (CTE)?

Third, brain injuries entail distinct temporal considerations. While some sports injuries can appear almost instantaneously (pulled hamstring) and some develop through repetitive strain (tennis elbow), medical science is currently unclear about the relative seriousness of single, traumatic brain assaults, compared to the long-term cumulative effect of lower force impacts. (Essentially, do both concussive injuries and sub-concussive impacts from heading footballs cause CTE?) Equally, while we tend to think of musculoskeletal injuries such as fractures as relatively problematic for ageing bodies which are often slower to physiologically repair, it is currently suggested that younger brains are more vulnerable (see, e.g. the discussion of SIS) and thus that injury can potentially lead to the most marked mental health problems amongst children. The dilemma then is in linking event with symptom manifestation. Does every impact cause incremental degradation of the brain?

To conclude, the brain is essential, distinctive, and complex, and these factors fuel a broader epistemic issue; how can we rationally respond to something if we don't know what it is? Chapter 4 revealed a range of issues in concussion science that are unresolved. We do not know if there is a period during which the brain is especially vulnerable, whether successive blows compound initial head injuries, or whether there is a relationship between either of these things and how long initial symptoms are manifest (McNamee et al. 2015). As we have no clear conceptualization of concussion, our diagnoses, incidence rates, etc., cannot be reliable. And yet, without injury audits, epidemiological surveys, or hospital admissions data (however flawed), how do we assess the scale of any potential longer-term harm? How could we, for instance, compare the relative risk of developing osteoarthritis or dementia as a consequence of participating in sport? Intuitively many would say that dementia would be a 'worse' condition to have (hence the prominence of CTE in popular cultural representations of the concussion crisis), but this is a socially constructed set of beliefs (see Chapter 8), attributed to all brain-related conditions. Ethical considerations are therefore complicated by issues about the certainty of the knowledge on which the response to concussion is based.

An institutional response to scientific uncertainty

These underlying scientific uncertainties ultimately generate new ethical dilemmas. For instance, considerations of whether there exists a distinction between 'simple' and 'complex' concussions, whether particular athletes are equipped to RTP more rapidly, or the lack of confidence in the diagnostic reliability of the SCAT tool (such that it is not recommended as a standalone method of assessment), compound the uncertainties consensus statements are designed to resolve. Most obviously and most problematically, there is an inherent contradiction in a group of experts seeking to make authoritative pronouncements, yet ultimately deferring to the individual judgement of those in the field of practice. If the leading biomedical researchers defer to those with practical experience, how 'expert' should we assume their knowledge to be? And if we are going to defer to experiential knowledge, why do the consensus statements solely defer to doctors' experiential knowledge rather than that developed by athletes, coaches, etc.? (See Chapter 8.)

Most particularly, because such marked scientific uncertainty exists in relation to CTE, it is highly ironic that the consensus statements are 'arguably the most authoritative proponents of CTE scepticism' (McNamee et al. 2015: 197). There are three main implications of the existing Concussion in Sport Group (CISG) position. First, the particular formulation appears to place mere participation in contact sports ('exposure') on a par with the incidence of concussion as potential causal factors. This appears contradictory to the placement of these discussions in the section titled 'special populations'. It further seems to divert attention away from suggestions that many find intuitively appealing: specifically, the idea that certain short-term symptoms (e.g. loss of consciousness) are particularly likely to be linked to the subsequent development of CTE. Second, it advocates that in the absence of a causal link, no action should be taken. This is both at odds with many of the CISG's pronouncements on concussion (for causal evidential links are often noticeably absent) and indeed contrary to a great deal of medicine in general, and neurology in particular. The reality of medicine is that such evidential certainty rarely exists (McNamee et al. 2015). Third, given the absence of certainty elsewhere in this field, it seems somewhat arbitrary to adopt a 'first do no harm' principle in relation to many SRC proscriptions (e.g. graduated RTP for asymptomatic individuals), yet reject such caution in relation to what is potentially the most serious concern of all.

The treatment of CTE in the concussion statements raises a final ethical issue in relation to concussion science: the way in which knowledge is mobilized and how it amplifies or de-amplifies social concern. Clear from the review in Chapter 4, there is relatively little that can be regarded as unequivocally right or wrong in this field. The most recent consensus statement of the American Medical Society for Sports Medicine (AMSSM) grades the level of evidence for its various recommendations. It contains no statements supported by 'consistent, good quality, patient-oriented evidence', ten points reflecting 'inconsistent or limited quality, patient-oriented evidence', and 26 recommendations below this threshold (Harmon et al. 2019).

However, if we explore two extreme examples we can at least see that there may be some more and relatively less judicious uses of concussion science. For instance, and particularly in relation to estimates of the prevalence of concussion, certain groups and individuals may have interests that align with a more conservative stance: highlighting the higher end of estimates, which might lead to social concern over concussion becoming more pronounced, the dedication of greater financial resource, and the enhanced status of concussion researchers within their scientific communities. This perhaps explains the CISG's difficult relationship with vested interests. While I am not aware of any specific examples of such behaviour, the potential for such positioning can be seen in the polar opposite behaviour, and the actions of the NFL's Mild Traumatic Brain Injury Committee (mTBIC) in submitting articles to *Neurology* journal which, taken together, have been interpreted as an attempt at 'denial' (Fainaru-Wada and Fainaru 2013). This latter set of actions also speaks to a duty of candour (or openness) which we see in relation governance and regulation. These ethical considerations are explored in the next section.

Governance and regulation

Broad social acceptance of the moral authority of biomedical science creates an expectation that the CISG will directly inform the regulation of concussion. But in addition to the concerns expressed about the scientific and clinical merit of some aspects of the consensus statements, it has also been argued that the process by which they are developed is problematic (see Chapter 4). While such concerns do not negate the view that the input of physicians in the regulation of concussion is necessary, equally they show that biomedical science alone is insufficient. Concussion is, as Greenhow and East (2015: 70) note, a 'wicked problem', 'one that is complex, difficult to define, evolving and has many interdependencies and many stakeholders'. In the penultimate section of this chapter we return to the role of the medical profession in the day-to-day regulation of concussion, but first we look at: 1) the ethical obligations on governing bodies of sport to take the lead on concussion; 2) the ethical issues raised by increased medical regulation; and 3) debates surrounding the prohibition of certain activities.

The obligations of sports governing bodies

In most of the sports affected by the concussion crisis (boxing, with its multiple world/international councils/associations/federations is an exception), we can identify a single governing body that can be described as a *dominant self-regulator*, possessing 'the exclusive ability to grant licences and rights to participate in the competition, and the power to design, implement and enforce policies, rules and laws of the game' (Greenhow and East 2015: 67). While there are different compensation and litigation cultures in different countries, and variations between governing bodies (such as the NFL, the AFL, and FIFA) in terms of jurisdictional scope, economic models, etc., generally such bodies operate in a regulatory space characterized by relative autonomy from direct governmental and legal influence. Indeed, self-regulation is seen as the most legitimate, effective, and efficient way to govern sport. For instance, remarkably stringent surveillance measures (e.g. the anti-doping system requiring athletes to inform the authorities of their 'where-abouts' for one hour every day to facilitate no-notice out-of-competition testing) are required for sports governing bodies to police the pharmacological intake of participants. Conversely, notions that sports participants make a voluntary assump-tion of risk enable physical contact in sports (a punch or tackle) which in other contexts would be deemed assault (Young 1993).

But equally, because the nature of sports participation is necessarily shaped by these governing bodies, the latter cannot simply 'wash their hands' and argue that adults are autonomous agents with sovereignty over their own actions. Rather, because sport governing bodies have ultimately set the parameters within which participants must act, they have a number of fundamental duties. For present pur-poses, the most notable of these are: 1) recognition of the salient issues (and if the governing body is ignorant, is it reasonable to expect it to be aware of the issues?); 2) sufficient representation of the risks; and 3) implementation of appropriate actions.

Scope of jurisdiction is also an important consideration in any governance issue. While the notion of public interest is always an imprecise concept (Greenhow and Gowthorp 2017), it does seem to be assumed by governing bodies which explicitly recognize their jurisdiction over participants at all levels of the sport (such as World Rugby) and/or explicitly state that player safety is a priority (e.g. the AFL). But it is equally, if perhaps more implicitly, relevant to those like the NFL whose direct influence is 'merely' a professional league, because of: 1) the social influence of those leagues; 2) expectations about the social benefits of sports participation (in relation to physical/mental health, 'character', etc.); and 3) a perceived 'trickle down' or 'ripple' effect from the mediated representation of elite athletes who are positioned as role models (Greenhow and East 2015; Orchard 2015). Each of the aforementioned governing bodies are effectively custodians of not just sports but important social institutions. Consequently, their duty is not just to maximize safety and minimize risk for the benefit of participants, but also to consider the potential cost burden to families, healthcare systems, and society more generally. In reality this duty of care frequently intermingles with a desire to protect the reputation of the individual sport (which translates into popularity, participation, sponsorship and media income). These two drivers do not always produce equally ethical outcomes (McNamee et al. 2015).

As we saw in Chapter 3, failure to exercise these duties or calls for further or different regulation becomes particularly pronounced where legal challenges are mounted. However, a sense that the NFL had fallen 'short of community and government expectations' led Congress to intervene and the subsequent inquiry criticized the league, 'for failing to regulate its sport for and in the best interests of its players and the public' (Greenhow and East 2015: 75, 76). The actions of the league (rule changes, commissioning research, etc.) were designed to enable it to be seen to engage in open self-regulation permeable to community, stakeholder, and, most importantly, government expectations. Moreover, the NFL litigation alerted other sports governing bodies to the potential liabilities of not fulfilling their obligations or duties of care, candour (or openness), and diligence (the duty to seek out relevant information) (Anderson nd). The regulatory convergence with the recommendations of the CISG is evidence of the former, while the implementation of injury surveillance systems and other research programmes is indicative of the latter. In relation to the duty of candour, it is not uncommon to see data from these injury audits regularly feature in medical journals and press releases, but as discussed in Chapter 7, there is a broader politics of knowledge to consider when these surveys are represented in the public domain.

Medical regulatory interventions

Given these fundamental duties and the threat of legal enforcement, much of what governing bodies have done to regulate concussion has been guided by a precautionary principle (Greenhow and East 2015). Consequently, as we saw in Chapter 3, many sports have changed their rules so as to reduce the risk of harm to the head. But critics might note that the implementation of a range of harm reduction policies has frequently entailed unintended consequences that raise additional ethical problems. While all major collision and contact sports now operate concussion exclusion rules (i.e. policies for the mandatory removal from play of those considered to be concussed), media coverage continually exposes instances where implementation is either questionable or clearly infringed. Indicatively, a systematic review of video footage of the 2014 FIFA World Cup tournament concluded that (at most) concussion assessment protocols were followed in just 37 per cent of cases of head collision (Cusimano et al. 2017).

Other regulations introduced in line with this precautionary principle include extended concussion assessment periods (to relieve the time pressures on clinicians) and compensatory substitution arrangements. These responses may, however, lead to different sorts of rule infringement or unethical behaviour as teams seek to capitalize on the opportunities they present (e.g. feigning head injury to either rest a player or retain the option for their return). Barry O'Driscoll, one of International Rugby Union's leading doctors, felt compelled to resign over the introduction of the head injury assessment protocols, arguing that they would inevitably lead to less conservative concussion management (effectively giving concussed players extra time to recover and therefore extend the opportunities to resume play). Some suspected that the Liverpool goalkeeper, Loris Karius, belatedly had himself diagnosed with concussion to provide mitigating evidence for a poor performance in the 2018 Champions' League final that threatened to see his club terminate his contract. Additionally, Orchard (2015) notes that the unlimited use of substitutes in the NFL appears to have enabled players to train to build strength rather than stamina and that the increased impact forces that result may be responsible for the relatively high incidence of concussion in the game. A similar case has been made in relation to protective clothing and risk compensation. Helmets may, in practice, become used as weapons, and boxing gloves may simply enable participants to inflict harder and more frequent blows on opponents (Sheard 2003).

Thus, ethical concerns lead us to question whether the conservative management of concussion necessarily reduces harm. Precautionary protocols may simply create an environment in which new opportunities to gain competitive advantages through unethical behaviour become available. They may ultimately increase the overall risk of injury to players. Consequently, regulation alone is not enough for a sport governing body to discharge its duty of care. Indeed, there have been frequent accusations that the processes for monitoring concussion regulations are too weak (Partridge 2014). Furthermore, sports governing bodies not only need to be transparent in ensuring fairness (comparable, say, to the clearly articulated drug testing regimes in sport) but must be seen to be effectively implementing regulations and punishing transgressions. This is particularly the case when we factor in the broader public interest remit of these bodies, for those playing at amateur levels (with voluntary officials and little or no trained healthcare provision) are unlikely to adopt and comply with harm reduction policies if elite players appear to circumvent concussion protocols.

Prohibition

In light of ongoing rule changes, Partridge and Hall (2014) consider what threshold of proof should be required to invoke such regulatory change. A key problem in this regard is that, as dominant self-regulators, sports governing bodies are often owners of the most comprehensive data sets or the gate-keepers to data gathering. Cantu and Hyman (2012), for instance, are critical of the Pop Warner League's previous failure to facilitate research, and Pollock (2014) makes similar claims about the rugby union authorities in the UK. It is on a similar basis that Goldberg (2013) concludes that while the NFL continues to refuse to make public all the historical data they have regarding concussion in the sport, the public will be denied an effective model of deliberative democracy, for a full and exhaustive public debate requires the free and reciprocal exchange of information.

The ethical arguments against external intervention – and at its extreme, prohibition – centrally revolve around 'agent sovereignty' and the belief that, ideally, people should be self-directing (Lopez Frias and McNamee 2017). JS Mill's *On Liberty* proposes that restrictions can only be justified if actions harm *others*, for self-harm is the prerogative of all individuals except 'idiots or infants'. It is on this basis that: 1) concussion exclusion rules are broadly supported, for by its very nature, concussion can entail the individual's reduced cognitive function (concussed athletes effectively become 'idiots'); and 2) greater regulation of children's sport can be justified. In both cases there is an ethical justification for others to act paternalistically.

Counter to this, Corlett (2014) has argued that college football should be banned because the potentially excessive costs of future healthcare cannot be justified. Similarly, Sailors (2015) supports prohibition, but on the grounds that people should be protected from their own actions if such actions entail the voluntary foregoing of future autonomy; in other words, the freedom to harm ourselves should not include self-harm to our future capacity to be free, such as selling oneself into slavery. But to argue for prohibition based on a cost to society which poses a sufficient/significant harm to *others* requires a demonstration of both relatively excessive costs and relatively high risks. Compare this, for instance, the risk of smoking tobacco which, while widely discouraged, is rarely banned (for adults at least) except in places where others might be exposed to harmful smoke. Additionally, we must consider that any prohibition would necessarily entail a cost of enforcement including questions of who would enforce and at what opportunity cost. (For instance, would it be better to stop people playing certain sports or stop people from stealing?) Thus, to stop people taking part in activities on the basis that they do irreparable harm to their future selves requires an illustration that such action represents a proportionate cost to society and that damage is definite rather than probable, complete rather than partial, and outweighs the short-term benefits to the self. The latter is particularly difficult given the substantial sums of money elite athletes can make during even a short career. Any comprehensive cost-benefit analysis would rely on a problematic quantification of the unquantifiable (see Lopez Frias and McNamee 2017 for an overview and critique of these arguments).

Thus, the argument *against* the prohibition of particular sports/activities is that they impose a cost on individuals who could no longer take part in the activities they personally value and which may further create economic value. This appears a more robust rationale than arguing simply that the voluntary assumption of risk – a kind of 'bracketed morality' – applies in sport due to participants' recognition that this is not the 'real world' and that they implicitly and knowingly accept the risks involved (Fry 2017). At the polar opposite to prohibition is the school of thought that suggests that even existing RTP regulations are overly paternalistic because they limit the freedom of individuals – whose decision-making powers are not impaired – to exercise voluntary choice (Johnson et al. 2015).

Johnson et al. (2015) further see a relatively compelling rationale for the use of child/youth specific protocols and tests, longer rest periods, etc. While, as we have seen, the case for the protected status of children and adolescents centres upon their designation as a vulnerable and 'special population', there are some necessarily fairly arbitrary judgements that have to be made in setting particular age thresholds. Why should an 11-year-old head a football while a 13-year-old cannot body check in ice hockey? Why ban tackle football up to 14 years old, but allow children to box? Generally speaking, policies should adopt a task-oriented approach to competence to consent; that is to say, the more complex the task the less freedom is granted to a 'vulnerable' person (Johnson et al. 2015). But, the degree of paternalism over children's sport-related behaviour rests on the rather more debatable point of how difficult it is (for a child rather than an adult) to identify the symptoms and consequences of concussion. How significantly should age mediate considerations here? On the assumption that they are not cognitively impaired, what is the evidence that these decisions are *further* beyond the capacity of an 11-year-old or 14-year-old than they are for an adult?

Perhaps least controversial of all though is Lopez Frias and McNamee's rejection of the prohibition of particular sports in their entirety. As they conclude,

> it is a stretch to suggest that the choice to engage in the activities is so wrongful as to be … [the equivalent] of engaging in voluntary enslavement or so necessarily harmful as to justify prohibition, and the other personal, economic and social costs that would entail.
>
> *(Lopez Frias and McNamee 2017: 276).*

Medical practice

Whatever the scientific evidence, and however the regulatory framework is drawn up, the ethical issues related to concussion are often ultimately mediated by the healthcare personnel called upon to operationalize these proscriptions. The rationale for such 'soft' paternalistic acts is that we presume that the clinician is more competent than the players in assessing the degree of harm to the brain. Like different branches of medical science, different forms of medical practice entail context-specific ethical concerns. Claims to uniqueness tend to be overstated for sports medicine (Malcolm 2016), and the four key medical ethical principles of beneficence, non-maleficence, justice, and patient autonomy all still apply. But there is certainly a case to say that sports medicine ethics are peculiar, and in this final section we focus on three areas within sports medicine where such principles are more or less directly challenged: clinical responsibility; conflicts of interest; and patient autonomy.

Considering the practice context requires us to re-examine the fundamental question of *who* should take responsibility for implementing concussion regulations. From a medical ethical viewpoint this should be guided by the principles of the pursuit of the relief of suffering (beneficence) and 'first do no harm' (non-maleficence). Social expectations and consensus statements defer to the expert knowledge of medicine in general and the clinical judgement of physicians specifically. However, the value that is also placed on experiential knowledge in the management of concussion opens up a range of ethical questions. We know, for instance, that physiotherapists and sports trainers invariably spend much more time with athletes than do doctors, tend to have more sports-specific training, and often have greater occupational experience (Malcolm 2017), so at what point does the value of a general educational qualification (for the statements make no mention of sport-specific qualifications or concussion training) supersede intimate experiential knowledge of treating the individual? Concussion symptoms, it should be remembered, are relatively patient-specific, so a blanket deference to medicine may deprive the concussed athlete of *better* healthcare. Similar questions might be raised about the value of independent assessors/matchday doctors who, by definition, must have less intimate knowledge of the patient. Impartiality may equate to impersonal medicine because generic principles rather than individualized considerations are applied (McNamee et al. 2016).

There is an opposite but perhaps equally valid issue, however; frequently athletic trainers (and, to a lesser extent, physiotherapists) do not share medicine's commitment to health. Rather their role may more explicitly be to provide for 'running repairs' (Partridge 2014: 68). Consequently, they are likely to be less directly committed to the principle of 'first do no harm'. While empirical studies of sports medicine practice have consistently borne this out, it is also clear that physicians are not immune to such considerations (Malcolm 2017). Orchard (2015: 2), for instance, states that whilst it is relatively easy to ignore a 'win at all costs' mentality in the amateur sport setting, 'the practicality of making a concussion diagnosis is more difficult' in the competitive sport context. Fundamental to the question of *who* should have clinical responsibility, therefore, is the question of conflicts of interest.

In sports medicine it is often claimed that the traditional two-way patient-doctor relationship is replaced, and made more complicated, by the existence of a patient-doctor-team triad (McNamee et al. 2016). More formalized in some contexts than others (US legislation enables a doctor to act more explicitly in the interests of a college sports team that employs him/her than in the interests of the patient), these relationships create pressures in all competitive sport settings. The interests of the coach, who tends to be the most powerful person in such situations, do not necessarily converge with the longer-term health interests of the player. Compromises are made and risks taken. Regulators of sport, therefore, have an ethical duty to both educate coaches (as the Lystedt Law demands) and ensure that coaches comply with concussion policies (which is undermined by the frequent absence of monitoring). This applies as much to mass participation levels of sports as it does to the elite. Perhaps most problematically of all, while such conflicts of interest are a fundamental obstacle to the effective regulation of concussion, there are examples where chief medical officers of sports governing bodies have effectively denied that such conflicts of interest exist (Partridge 2014), and a general sense in which they are given insufficient emphasis in concussion regulation.

Finally, the practicalities of the medical management of concussion directly raise ethical issues about the autonomy of the patient. There are, of course, various times when patient autonomy is not possible, for example, when the patient is either physically or mentally unable to give informed consent. This could apply in any medical emergency situation. But in the context of concussion in sport, autonomy may be complicated by the self-belief of the 'patient' that they are coherent and unimpaired, the clinicians' experience that self-report is unreliable in these instances, and the regulatory requirements to act with caution. Indeed, the existence of any regulation effectively imposes a degree of coercion on the individual, and here it falls to the clinician to act as the enforcer. As a consequence of this, clinicians frequently report experiencing pressures from players who dispute their diagnoses or resist the rationale for a graduated return to play (RTP) (see Chapter 6). The universal adoption of graduated RTP protocols ultimately mean that the initial diagnosis, rather than symptom resolution, becomes the key issue (McNamee et al.

2016). The increased and time-sensitive pressures on clinicians may create conditions which encourage unethical medical practice (see previous section).

A potential response that clinicians may invoke to alleviate this pressure is
avoidance of diagnosis (Partridge 2014). Context and conflicts of interest are
important here. Thus, the avoidance response has both been alleged in some high
media profile cases and, as we shall see (Chapter 6), empirically illustrated in
behavioural science research. Avoidance has the additional benefit of allowing the
clinician to circumvent another potential ethical dilemma in the treatment of
concussion: the patient's right to confidentiality. Because concussion injuries have
specific regulations, and require athletes to undergo specific protocols prior to
returning to play, the normal right to confidentiality which patients hold must
effectively be waived. As concussion injuries are subject to a unique set of regulations, the concussed player must inevitably have their medical condition made
public. Moreover, the greater the level of transparency required to ensure compliance with concussion regulations the further the ethical principles of patient
autonomy and the right to confidentiality are undermined. There is an argument
therefore that constraints on participants' rights to confidentiality should be
informed by the practice community, though this is noticeably absent in sport at
present (McNamee et al. 2015).

Conclusion

This chapter has explored the ethical issues that arise in relation to the science,
governance and day-to-day medical management of concussion in sport. These
issues are numerous, wide-ranging and frequently intersect, and attempts to
remove or reduce ethical problems sometimes create new or additional dilemmas.
Highlighting these ethical issues enables us to develop a more holistic understanding of the concussion crisis in sport. These ethical issues both explain why
concussion creates such a high level of concern for sports authorities and sporting
publics and provide an essential basis on which to fully understand the actions
that have and may in future be taken. Ethical issues will inform our analysis in
Chapter 9, but our next task is to see how the ethical debates charted here
combine with the medical considerations discussed in Chapter 4 in the lived
experience of concussion. How do participants, coaches, and those clinicians
charged with implementing concussion management protocols experience sport's
concussion crisis?

References

Anderson, J. (no date) 'Concussion, sport and the law', www.sportsintegrityinitiative.com/
    concussion-sport-and-the-law/
Cantu, R. and Hyman, M. (2012) *Concussions and Our Kids*. Boston, MA: Mariner Books.
Corlett, J.A. (2014) 'Should inter-collegiate football be eliminated? Assessing the arguments
    philosophically', *Sport, Ethics and Philosophy*, 8(2): 116–136.

Cusimano, M., Casey, J., Jing, R. et al. (2017) 'Assessment of head collision events during the 2014 FIFA World Cup tournament', *Journal of the American Medical Association*, 317 (24): 2548–2549.

Fainaru-Wada, M. and Fainaru, S. (2013) *League of Denial*. New York: Crown Business.

Fry, J. (2017) 'Two kinds of brain injury in sport', *Sport, Ethics and Philosophy*, 11(3): 294–306.

Fry, J. and McNamee, M. (2017) 'Sport, ethics and neurophilosophy', *Sport, Ethics and Philosophy*, 11(3): 259–263.

Goldberg, D. (2013) 'Mild traumatic brain injury, the National Football League, and the manufacture of doubt: an ethical, legal, and historical analysis', *Journal of Legal Medicine*, 34 (2): 157–191.

Greenhow, A. and East, J. (2015) 'Custodians of the game: ethical considerations for football governing bodies in regulating concussion management', *Neuroethics*, 8: 65–82.

Greenhow, A. and Gowthorp, L. (2017) 'Head injuries and concussion issues', in N. Shulenkorf and S. Frawley (eds.), *Critical Issues in Global Sports Management*, Abingdon, UK: Routledge, 93–112.

Harmon, K., Clugston, J., Dec, K., et al. (2019) 'American Medical Society for Sports Medicine position statement: concussion in sport', *British Journal of Sports Medicine*, 53: 213–225.

Johnson Thornton, D. (2011) *Brain Culture: Neuroscience and Popular Media*. New Brunswick, NJ: Rutgers University Press.

Johnson, S., Partridge, B., and Gilbert, F. (2015) 'Framing the debate: concussion and mild traumatic brain injury', *Neuroethics*, 8: 1–4.

Lopez Frias, F. and McNamee, M. (2017) 'Ethics, brain injuries, and sports: prohibition, reform and prudence', *Sport, Ethics and Philosophy*, 11(3): 264–280.

Malcolm, D. (2016) 'Confidentiality in sports medicine', *Clinics in Sports Medicine*, 35: 205–215.

Malcolm, D. (2017) *Sport, Medicine and Health: The Medicalization of Sport?* London: Routledge.

McNamee, M., Partridge, B., and Anderson, L. (2015) 'Concussion in sport: conceptual and ethical issues', *Kinesiology Review*, 4: 190–202.

McNamee, M., Partridge, B., and Anderson, L. (2016) 'Concussion ethics and sports medicine', *Clinics in Sports Medicine*, 35(2): 257–268.

Mill, J.S. (1892) *On Liberty*. London: Longmans Green.

Orchard, J. (2015) 'Match of the decade: risk management of concussion versus high-speed collisions in the football codes', *Medical Journal of Australia*, 203(7): 1–2E1.

Partridge, B. (2014) 'Dazed and confused: sports medicine, conflicts of interest, and concussion management', *Bioethical Inquiry*, 11: 65–74.

Partridge, B. and Hall, W. (2014) 'Repeated head injuries in Australia's collision sports highlight ethical and evidential gaps in concussion management policies', *Neuroethics*, 8(1): 39–45.

Pollock, A. (2014) *Tackling Rugby: What Every Parent Should Know about Injuries*. London: Verso.

Sailors, P. (2015) 'Personal foul: an evaluation of the moral status of football', *Journal of the Philosophy of Sport*, 42(2): 269–286.

Sheard, K. (2003) 'Boxing in the western civilizing process', in E. Dunning, D. Malcolm, and I. Waddington (eds.), *Sport Histories: Figurational Studies of the Development of Modern Sports*, London: Routledge, 15–30.

Young, K. (1993) 'Violence, risk and liability in male sports culture', *Sociology of Sport Journal*, 10(4): 373–396.

6

CONCUSSION AND BEHAVIOURAL SCIENCE

Ash couldn't remember what had happened, but she could answer the physio's questions: 'Saturday. 3–0'. As the fog lifted and things became clearer, Ash realized the team couldn't lose another player. That's what coach would want. The physio would try to get her to come off, but who cared what they thought? 'If this is what it takes to play sport...'

The account of the concussion crisis we have seen so far has, in a sense, been largely one-sided. We have seen when, how, and why concussion became a social issue. We have seen the formalization of increasingly conservative medical guidelines for the management of sports-related concussion (SRC), and we have seen some of the governance and ethical debates unique to this field. But as crisis is fundamentally about imbalance – the conflict between different groups – we need to better understand the other side of this equation. Simply stated, the concussion crisis inherently involves the sport population's resistance to proposed change. If those active in sport simply heeded these precautionary messages and responded accordingly there would be no crisis to examine.

The reality, however, is that we see a marked disparity between the precautionary position evident in the wider society (and medical community) and the way participants perceive and behave in response to concussion. Consequently, this chapter looks at research which tells us more about the *lived experience* of concussion in sport. Specifically, how do various parties – players, coaches, and healthcare providers – actually behave when confronted with concussion? Most importantly, how does research conducted within the behavioural sciences *explain* this behaviour?

Responses to concussion injury

Despite important cross-sport and cross-cultural differences in the profile of concussion as a social issue (Chapter 3), research has continually positioned athletes as largely 'failing' to report their signs or symptoms of concussion. For instance, a study of combat sport participants found that 21 per cent endorsed concealing head injuries from coaches and medical staff, and 40 per cent had returned to training/ competition on the same day as incurring a head injury (Bennett et al. 2018). Similar studies have shown that 50.3 per cent of former NFL players (active from the 1940s to the 2000s) had sustained a head injury and not reported it to medical staff (Kerr et al. 2018), and 40 per cent of contemporary rugby players have manipulated a medical assessment for concussion (O'Connell and Molloy 2016).

Fraas et al.'s (2013) study of elite Irish rugby players adds further detail. Here, only about half (53.4 per cent) of those who had experienced at least one (suspected) concussion in the previous season had subsequently revealed their concerns to another person. Moreover, not infrequently, they had chosen to disclose this information to a friend or family member rather than one of the club's healthcare providers. Tellingly, not one of the players had disclosed their injury concerns directly to the person ultimately responsible for deciding who does/does not play or train (their coach). Furthermore, while a significant number of players had suspected their teammates of suffering from a concussion, most stated that they had not and would not intervene in such cases. This behaviour is persistent across time and studies. A more recent study of 350 international players drawn from 20 top rugby playing nations found that 28 per cent had concealed post-concussion symptoms in order to start the return to play (RTP) protocol.[1]

While the economic motivations of being a professional athlete must influence these behaviours, we also know that this behaviour is replicated across other levels of sporting performance. For instance, Delaney et al. (2002) established that approximately two-thirds of Canadian footballers and soccer players in college believed that they had been concussed during the previous year, that in excess of 80 per cent of these had experienced multiple concussions, and that around 20 per cent had endured symptoms for a day or longer. Their follow-up study utilizing a wider cohort of students participating *across* varsity sports found that while concussion incidence was lower (20 per cent) the vast majority (78.3 per cent), like their professional counterparts, had not sought medical attention (Delaney et al. 2015). Similarly, Sanderson et al.'s (2017) survey of the users of the US-based *pinkconcussions.com* advocacy website found that 78 per cent of male and 69 per cent of female respondents had played through a concussion without reporting it, while a study of high school athletes also identified the 'gross underreporting of recalled concussion events' (Register-Mihalik et al. 2013: 651). So well-established is this trend that Kroshus et al. (2015) list 11 such studies that chart the failure or underreporting of concussions among athletic populations and Mrazik et al. (2015) estimate that 'non-compliance' ranges between 25 per cent and 60 per cent of research subjects in the various sports surveyed. So endemic is this problem thought to be that a specific test – the Rosenbaum Concussion Knowledge and Attitudes Survey – is now widely used in this type of research (Rosenbaum and Arnett 2010).

The most frequently cited reasons for this behaviour are based around knowledge and commitment, with players: 1) either not knowing that they have been concussed or not believing their symptoms to be serious; and 2) deciding to continue participating either because they simply wanted to play on, or because they did not want to let their team mates down (Broglio et al. 2010). In addition to this, some cite the specific manifestation of the condition as significant, referring to concussion as an 'invisible' injury (Bloom et al. 2004). Over time, however, the idea that failure to report stems from a *lack* of knowledge has become steadily less credible. Williams et al.'s (2016) study of English professional soccer players' knowledge of and attitudes towards concussion showed a clear mismatch between understanding as expressed in the relatively detached context of a questionnaire survey and the real-life scenarios presented in interview. So while players could identify most of the common signs and symptoms of concussion, and would even express 'conservative concussion attitudes' in response to a survey (Williams et al. 2016: 201), they would *talk about* attempting to play through concussions, 'favourably' compare concussion to more 'serious' musculoskeletal injuries such as groin strains, and state how they would be inclined to take greater risks with their personal health if the match was particularly important or if a lack of available substitutes would mean withdrawal leaving their team at a competitive disadvantage. The precautionary guidelines about concussion were both *known* and *understood*, and indeed deemed *acceptable* when viewed in the abstract, but the footballers showed little commitment to their implementation when faced with real-life scenarios. Similarly, Kroshus et al.'s (2015: 69) study of NCAA athletes concluded that neither knowledge nor previous personal experience of concussion 'were significantly associated with reporting intention' (see also Chinn and Porter 2016), while a subsequent study (Kroshus et al. 2018) found that those with a prior diagnosis of concussion were *more likely* to continue playing when concussed. Clearly, then, behaviours are relatively impervious to the broader public concerns about concussion, and the associated increases in awareness of the potential short- and long-term health consequences of concussion injuries focussed on by the cultural industries.

Qualitative research provides more stark illustrations of how athletes respond to concussion. Caron et al.'s (2013) study of retired NHL players showed that even after some years outside the sport, concussion injuries were seen as routine or simply a workplace hazard. Some recalled playing games where their vision or balance was severely affected. So frequent were concussion injuries that interviewees often could not quantify the number of incidences they had experienced through their careers. Hiding symptoms from teammates, coaches, and medical staff was presented as a common course of action.

This acceptance continued despite respondents' experiences of concussion symptoms which were wide-ranging (from pain to mood alteration), severe (including disruption of daily living and even suicidal ideation), and long-term (lasting up to 14 years). Yet at the same time, somewhat ambiguous attitudes were expressed about how directly specific conditions were the consequence of concussion, with some wondering whether the symptoms they experienced were simply part of the ageing process. The physiological experience of concussion was compounded by the emotional turmoil created by uncertainty over the condition (e.g. how long symptoms would last, the potential that one might be 'losing one's mind') and the withdrawal and isolation fostered by concussion management protocols (see Chapter 4). Coaches often did little to counteract the effects of isolation and, in extreme cases, sought to exacerbate loneliness as a strategy for encouraging more rapid RTP (see Roderick et al. 2000 for a discussion of such practices in sport).

Caron et al.'s (2013) study also leads us to rethink the degree of emphasis placed on the idea that concussion is unique in being an 'invisible' injury. Rather than being defined in dualistic visible-invisible terms, it is more accurate to conceive of all injuries as existing on a spectrum of visibility. For instance, many fractures cannot be seen without the use of x-ray, and athletes frequently undergo MRI scans to diagnose soft tissue injuries. Concussion may be *more* 'invisible' in the sense that it is not amenable to contemporary diagnostic imaging techniques, but in many other respects the signs and symptoms (disorientation, confusion, loss of consciousness) are clearly detectable, to both the individual concerned and those around them. While concussions can certainly be concealed in many instances, again so can other sports injuries. The frequent finding that athletes both suspect their teammates of carrying concussions and would be reluctant to bring their actions to the attention of coaches and medical staff (e.g. Sye et al. 2006; Fraas et al. 2013) illustrates how easy it is for people to (think they can) diagnose concussion. Thus, the key issue is not (in)visibility but (un)certainty, and how this creates a peculiar set of *attitudes towards* concussion. The clear mismatch between the perceived effects and subsequent (lack of) behavioural change seems simply irrational to those lobbying for change and is thus a key dynamic in sport's concussion crisis.

The influence of social relations

To challenge this sense of irrationality and provide a more adequate explanation of the 'under-reporting problem' we need to locate these behaviours in the broader set of social relations. For instance, Kroshus et al. (2014) draw on the 'theory of planned behaviour' which predicts that performed behaviour stems from attitude, perceived social norms and perceived ability to perform a behaviour. Elsewhere they consider the use of 'social cognitive theory', in which individual psychology, environmental factors, and behaviour interact to create a form of 'reciprocal determinism', or a feedback loop between the responses of significant others (often coaches) and concussion reporting behaviours (Kroshus et al. 2015: 67). Similarly, Sanderson et al. (2017: 272) invoke the idea of 'muted group theory', arguing that the dominant group is able to establish the 'rules and systems of accepted discourse' to suppress alternative perspectives. Briefly stated, in the context of contact team sports, the valorization of masculinity as expressed through tolerance of pain and injury prevents athletes from expressing concerns about the physical impact of concussion on health.

These studies usefully direct our attention to the pressures brought through social relations. They connect with research findings that show that coaches struggle to distinguish the signs and symptoms of concussion from other conditions and harbour misconceptions about the medical management of concussion (Mrazik et al. 2015). Indicatively, the support players received is very varied, with some coaches making decisive interventions to precipitate retirement, and others apparently entirely disregarding this particular type of injury (Caron et al. 2013; Sye et al. 2006). Kroshus et al. (2015) further explored four different sources of support/ pressure – teammates, coaches, parents, and fans – and found that 25 per cent of collegiate athletes perceived themselves to have experienced pressure to play while suffering from concussion from at least one of these sources. Pressure was relatively evenly spread across the four groups, and there were slight (but not statistically significant) variations in the pressures felt by male and female athletes. However, those that experienced *all four sources* of pressure concurrently were the most likely to express an intention to continue playing when incurring future head injuries. While a recognized limitation of this study is the lack of data on the intensity or duration of pressure, the notion of pressure highlights the significance of social relations and logically leads us towards more culturally oriented explanations.

The relative merits of such an approach are evident in studies that compare the reasons for gendered differences in reporting behaviour. For instance, Colón et al. (2017) found that female college students tended to have fewer concussions, but a more elongated post-concussion RTP. Similarly, O'Connell and Molloy (2016: 522, 527) state that 'female players respond less favourably to concussion than male players', are more likely to worry about the longer-term effects, and exhibit 'the potential for poorer recovery'. The gendered assumptions that inform studies such as O'Connell and Molloy (2016) feed into the CISG consensus statement (Chapter 4), where the apparently more cautious behaviour of females is effectively defined as deviant from the male norm even though, as we can see here, the behaviour of male athletes is widely perceived to itself be problematic.

In seeking to explain such differences, Sanderson et al. (2017: 267) argue that alignment to 'sport cultural norms' is a gendered process. Drawing on the broader sociological literature on pain and injury in sport, they suggest that these norms consist of two subthemes – the pain principle and team allegiance – and attribute the non-reporting of concussions to these familiar explanations – essentially knowledge, perceived severity, and commitment – plus a perceived lack of resources (i.e. healthcare support). However, they further conclude that females' non-reporting is more likely to be driven by the perceived lack of resources, a belief that their injuries are not particularly severe, and subcultural expectations around continuing to play whilst in pain. Conversely, male concussion reporting behaviour is more likely to be driven by notions of team allegiance. Ultimately then, male and female athletes' different concussion behaviours derive from their different subcultural norms.

The wider sociological research on pain and injury in sport is indeed an important resource in understanding athletes' disregard of the risks of head injury.

Broadly speaking, this research shows that the patterns of behaviour described previously are subculturally *normal*. Regardless of type of injury, athletes exhibit a remarkably high tolerance towards experiences of pain and injury; athletes tend to carry on training for, and competing in, their sport despite an awareness of underlying injury problems; and athletes experience various forms of pressure from significant others which leads them to normalize and accept these culturally specific ways of behaving. The explanations most frequently presented to understand these phenomena are:

1. The 'sport ethic' (Hughes and Coakley 1991), expressed through an unquestioning commitment to the norms of performance sport, particularly ideas about athletes' dedication, distinction, resilience, and non-defeatism;
2. The 'masculinity and sport' nexus (Messner 1992), in which sport provides a social context where violence is 'naturalized' as a male characteristic. This, in turn, facilitates a specific contextual morality in which inflicting and receiving pain and injury is deemed both normal and legitimate (for males); and
3. Structural explanations exemplified by Nixon's (1992) concept of the 'sportsnet', in which a specific network of relationships (typically concentrating on athletes, coaches, medical personnel, owners, fans, etc.) entails the displacement of risk such that a relatively small group (athletes) carry the entire responsibility for the broader organization's success/failure and are thus encouraged to undertake high-risk behaviours.

To a greater or lesser extent each of these ideas can be applied to understand concussion-related behaviours. While the notion of masculinity could explain why females seem to take longer to recover from concussion, it is counter intuitive to studies which show a higher incidence of concussion among males. This partly reflects trends in the wider field which question whether gender is a very significant mediator of injury behaviour (see, e.g. Young and White 1993) and requires further exploration. Most particularly, concussion behaviours do seem to resonate with Hughes and Coakley's (1991) ideas about commitment and culturally specific norms.

But while concussion related behaviours conform to a broad subcultural pattern of responses to sports injury, we must not neglect the specificity of concussion as a condition. For instance, Colón et al.'s (2017) 'cultural domain analysis' of college students' descriptions of the consequences and effects of concussion identified three main clusters of terms: physical/body (fatigue, nausea, pain, headache); mind/brain (confusion, dizzy, balance, blurred vision, concentration); and severe (trauma, brain injury, memory loss). In subsequent interviews the students began by emphasizing musculoskeletal elements (bruised, rattled, etc.) but became more hesitant and less coherent when they tried to articulate the cognitive and emotional dimensions of concussions that are related to the mind/brain. Consequently, it appeared that athletes' perceptions of head injuries 'seem heavily influenced by the more prevalent cultural understanding of sport injuries as skeletomuscular' (Colón et al.

2017: 1085). Colón et al.'s findings relate both with the discussion of neuroscience ethics in Chapter 5 and with interview data with amateur rugby union players in Ireland (Liston et al. 2018). Here, players explicitly made comparisons between musculoskeletal and cerebral injuries and, despite some knowledge regarding the potential dangers, stated their clear preference for receiving the latter.

This hierarchy of injury concerns – fundamentally at odds with broader cultural industry's representation of sport's concussion crisis – can, however, be explained by the functional criteria by which sports injuries tend to be evaluated (Malcolm and Sheard 2002; Sanderson et al. 2017). Simply stated, because physical pain is such an ever-present feature of participation in competitive combat, collision, and contact sports, participants find it more meaningful and socially useful to only define as injuries those physical conditions which evidently limit or disable their ability to function effectively within the sport. The apparent unwillingness of sports participants to modify the risks they take in relation to head injuries (i.e. playing on, not seeking medical attention) stems partly from the belief that concussion injuries tend not, or tend only temporarily, to restrict one from functioning on the field of play. While, as we saw in relation to the retired NHL players, post-concussion symptoms can last for years, more commonly they last for a much shorter period of time than, for example, a muscle tear might. This helps explain the explicitly 'irreverent' attitude towards concussion many sports participants express including attempts to 'work the system', 'lie to yourself', or 'bluff your way through' on-field diagnostic assessment (Liston et al. 2018: 675). When we talk about function here, we do so in the sense that function will always be socially evaluated.

Thus, in terms of functionality, a distinct feature of SRC is that it evokes a qualitatively distinct form of uncertainty. Uncertainty has been deployed in the sociology of medicine to understand a wide range of 'patient' experiences (Fox 2000). It may stem from the peculiar physical sensations which people feel they need assistance to resolve, but particularly from the kind of open-ended and unbounded potential impact of an injury/illness on one's broader life expectations (the latter termed existential uncertainty). For athletes, this uncertainty is likely to focus on their ability to function in sport and retain their position within sports subcultures. While concussed players 'experience uncertainty because their bodies feel unusual, . . . they seldom experience problems which they themselves cannot resolve and rarely, or only briefly, experience uncertainty in the form of concern about sporting performance' (Malcolm 2009: 200). Consequently, the motivation to report injuries and seek medical help is reduced. The apparent 'failure' of athletes to do so can thus largely be attributed to the relative *lack* of existential uncertainty concussion patients tend to experience/perceive.

An additional and important part of the decision-making equation is the sense of value participants attach to playing sport. Behavioural scientists researching sport have for many years talked about the identity-defining character of the activity. For those who regularly engage in sport, these activities become one of the central elements of the way in which they understand themselves, structure their relations, and give meaning to their place in the social world. In line with this, the interviewees in Colón et al.'s (2017) study described a wide range of negative consequences that enforced withdrawal from sport could entail. Some envisaged themselves being devastated or inconsolable if forced to stop playing sport. The perceived psycho-social benefits of sports participation included the replacement of family bonds disrupted by the transition to college/adulthood and the construction of new group identities. Sport was also variously seen as an important source of positive mental health, enabling students to cope with the stresses and challenges of academic life. These statements correlate with the broader ideology of sport in contemporary Western societies (see Chapter 8). Indeed, the strong sense of personal autonomy which athletes exhibit is likely in part to stem from the sense of social validation for participating in sport more generally. This partly explains why athletes think it is justifiable for individuals to make their own RTP decisions after incurring a concussion (Williams et al. 2016).

The role and behaviour of clinicians

To this point the focus has primarily been upon the athletes themselves. The overriding implication – indeed the core assumption in the literature – has been that it is *their* behaviour – the '*gross*' underreporting (Register-Mihalik et al. 2013), the knowledge '*deficit*' (O'Connell and Molloy 2016) – that is problematic, and that others around them either facilitate or are powerless to 'correct' this behaviour. Implicit in these accounts, therefore, is a sense that the primary failing of medicine is to be absent or lack influence.

This assumption is, however, contradicted by the existing research on the behaviour of healthcare providers in sport. For instance, family physicians and other healthcare providers exhibit misconceptions and variable treatment practices which in part stem from sometimes working with outdated information (Mrazik et al. 2015). Surveys evidence the limited training of Canadian medical students, and that a third of American paediatric neurologists believe that they have not been adequately trained to deal with concussions (Mrazik et al. 2015). While Mathieu et al. (2018: 1) argued that although 'major gaps' in the concussion education delivered in Canadian medical schools had been addressed, 'persistent deficiencies in a minority of schools' remain.

The situation is similar within *sports* medicine. A survey of professional soccer club medical officers in England found that 'only 21% of teams routinely record an approved preseason cognitive score . . . only 42% complete the appropriate post-concussion assessment, and . . . a quarter of club doctors had no knowledge of the operant consensus statement' (Price et al. 2012: 1000). Similarly, retired NHL players reported an increased sense of isolation when sourcing medical attention because 'no one understood' their condition/experience, while others considered themselves 'unfortunate' that the reporting of a concussion incident meant that medical staff insisted on more conservative injury management on subsequent occasions (Caron et al. 2013). It cannot be assumed that clinicians' knowledge is either perfect or implemented in consistent ways. There is, in other words, a need to 'identify the disparity between the public and paradigmatic promises of medicine and the private problems of practice' (Malcolm 2018: 146).

Again, recourse to the wider sociology of sport literature can guide our understanding. While relatively underdeveloped compared to the literature on athletes' responses to pain and injury, research on the working practice of sport clinicians has shown that medical provision in sport varies considerably. For instance, a survey of English rugby union clubs found that less than a quarter were compliant with regulations regarding the provision of medical personnel and facilities (Wing et al. 2018). Although at the elite end of sport huge resources are committed to enable the team's most valuable 'assets' to remain 'productive', more typically athletes rely on minimal, often voluntary, medical cover provided by people who may not have sport-specialist skills (or indeed may have only minimal medical qualifications) or be able to devote much time to the cause (Malcolm 2017). This is particularly the case in female sport (Kotarba 2012) as reflected by the gendered responses noted earlier. The medical provision in sport 'is highly fragmented, of very variable quality and ultimately is frequently retarded more by the traditions and culture of sport than by limited financial resources' (Malcolm 2017: 117).

Specifically, for this *applied* form of medicine (as opposed to the 'pure' medical science that was charted in Chapter 4), practitioners lack autonomy, may be relatively isolated from professional colleagues, and are ultimately highly dependent on their clients. Indeed, such 'applied' sports medicine bears many of the hallmarks of the 'everyday work settings' (Freidson 1970) in which clinicians are *least able* to assert authority and will most likely be influenced by lay evaluations of 'appropriate' treatment. Most frequently the challenges clinicians experience in this context relate to balancing the fundamental ethical commitment of medicine to the enhancement of human health against the performance-orientation of sport and the degree to which this is complicated by the doctor-patient-coach triad in sport (see Chapter 5). While the balance of commitment has been shown to vary across contexts – from athletes at college (Safai 2003; Walk 1997), state-sponsored national representatives pursuing Olympic medals (Theberge 2007; Scott 2012), and employed by professional sports teams (Waddington 2000; Malcolm 2006) – at its 'weakest' clinicians are always conscious of their need to advocate precaution as a counter to the more pervasive culture of risk. At its 'strongest' and at the highest levels of sport, clinicians recognize that risk/performance is the default position (Theberge 2007).

Compounding factors include the commercial pressures that link sport performance with revenue with clinicians' job security and pay (Anderson and Jackson 2012), but more universally clinicians identify the importance of negotiating with their clients (both coaches and athletes) to ensure they continue to have the access to practice. Various studies have shown that the relative dominance of coaches in sport can mean that clinicians experience reduced clinical autonomy with diagnoses compromised, the time frame for RTP contested, and players frequently rejecting and undermining clinical expertise through the use of their own lay medical knowledge and through a practice of 'therapist hopping'. In some cases, clinicians become the 'tools' of management and have been shown to act unethically in coercing athletes to forego their own interests (i.e. health) for the sake of the team (Waddington 2000).

Drawing on this body of work, a study of concussion management in English rugby union demonstrates how patterns of regulatory non-compliance and a lack of standardized concussion protocol implementation (as noted previously) are shaped by the networks of relations in which sports clinicians are embedded (Malcolm 2009). So strong are these relations that they influence the social construction of their medical knowledge and practice. More specifically, the study highlighted how practice in relation to concussion was constrained by two forms of uncertainty: 1) epistemological uncertainty, or clinicians' awareness of the limited nature of the medical understanding of concussion; and; 2) clinical uncertainty, or clinicians' lack of conviction in their own grasp of both the appropriate diagnosis and treatment of concussion. Clinicians noted how issues related to concussion brought them into the most significant cases of conflict they ever experienced with either players who resented the curtailment of their activities for a condition which they felt was not limiting their performance (and thus the *lack* of existential uncertainty; for examples, see Caron et al. 2013 and Colón et al. 2017), and the coaches who were unconvinced that they should be deprived of the services of seemingly asymptomatic players. Consequently, clinicians had embarked on projects to investigate the 'pure' concussion science but had found contradictions and incoherence in the broader literature. They used these findings as a rationale to legitimate their own clinical limitations but went further in citing the specific constraints experienced in this particular practice context. Dehydrated players, lack of time to assess, and the relatively routine expression of a set of symptoms which were, moreover, not necessarily distinct to the condition were all cited as factors that served to complicate the 'applied' science of concussion management, but actually these were the *consequence* of clinicians' uncertainty rather than the root cause.

Ultimately, clinicians were disinclined to implement diagnostic and treatment guidelines in the 'spirit' of the regulatory statements, but chose instead to follow the explicit wording which gave primacy to individual clinical judgement (see Chapter 4). Effectively this meant that they were able to act in ways which reduced conflict with those around them and therefore improved patient compliance. They adopted their own paradigms to understand concussion, seeking to avoid an 'official' or formal diagnosis of concussion wherever possible, and giving primacy to loss of consciousness as a diagnostic sign. This became central partly because it was both the most evident and non-negotiable sign, but equally because it was what others perceived to be the most severe symptom and thus took as acceptable grounds for intervention (see e.g. Sye et al. 2006). Clinicians further developed personal treatment philosophies which drew on their individual, experiential knowledge of the individual players, incorporating both a player's prior incidence of concussion and previous patterns of recovery and thus foregrounded the ability of the affected individual to function in their sporting role. Through these working practices, clinicians demonstrated a closer allegiance to the norms of the sporting subculture in which their 'applied' science was practiced than to the 'pure' scientific discipline that formed the basis of their professional status. Ultimately, the degree of uncertainty about concussion was so great that it created the conditions for social pressures to exert a particularly strong influence on medical treatment. Almost invariably this led to the less, rather than more, conservative management of concussion (Malcolm 2009).

While the greater public awareness of concussion and a greater knowledge of its various symptoms and longer-term potential harm might lead us to expect that this particular dynamic between professional- and lay-medical knowledge will change over time, a subsequent study of the experiences of soccer club clinicians in the English professional leagues produced remarkably similar findings (Malcolm 2017; 2018). Fifteen years on, the inconsistencies in concussion diagnosis and evaluation remained, with doctors and physiotherapists expressing their sense of confusion and deploying redundant distinctions between 'minor' and 'major' concussions. Indicatively, they reported very variable descriptions of rates of incidence, from every few games to every few years (see the discussion of epidemiology in Chapter 4). Evidence was found of both external pressures being put on clinicians to modify their diagnoses and prognoses, and regulatory non-compliance as the 'fudging' or blurring of clinical judgements is driven by concerns to avoid conflict with their patients. Once again, clinicians' understanding of concussion seemed to be shaped as much by the views of the 'clients' they served as it did by the scientific understanding set out in biomedical consensus statements and reflected in sport regulations.

There may be four reasons for such continuity. First, this behaviour stems from the ongoing biomedical scientific uncertainty over concussion. Specifically, as we have seen (Chapter 4), while increasingly standardized and formalized in recent years, concussion science has neither significantly enhanced our understanding of the underlying mechanisms of the injury, nor developed more sophisticated diagnostic tools. Consequently, management guidelines remain rooted in a rather weak evidential base. Second, the rate of change in concussion management protocols further confuses clinicians (Mrazik et al. 2015) and leaves them implementing outdated procedures or simply uncertain of their own compliance. Allied to this, the traditional status and authority of medicine – as an inscrutable profession and practice – means that there is relatively little if any monitoring of clinicians' work within sport (compare, for instance, the number of studies which focus on participants' 'underreporting' with those examining clinicians' imperfect working practices). Fourth, the continued deference to individual clinical judgement, while necessary given the degree of epistemological uncertainty regarding concussion, ultimately facilitates the influence of non-medical criteria. In these particular sporting contexts, the result is that performance and functionality tend to take priority over considerations of players' health. Thus, if players want to, and if they say that they are fit to play on despite exhibiting some signs and symptoms of concussion, they are likely to be able to. Medical personnel may be unable, but equally at times *reluctant*, to stop them.

Conclusion

Through this chapter we have seen the propensity of concussed athletes to dis-regard signs and symptoms and continue to take part in sport contrary to medical and regulatory stipulations. We have further seen how relations with significant others frequently serve to reinforce such attitudes, and we have explored the all-consuming nature of sports subcultures which are sometimes influential enough to shape the practice and even the *knowledge* of clinicians. The attitudinal imbalance that forms the core of sport's concussion crisis is thus, on this side at least, deeply culturally embedded.

It is worth concluding with some reflections on the empirical studies that have largely informed this chapter. Three things are particularly striking. First, a concept frequently implicit but at times also explicit in this work is the notion of 'undiag-nosed concussions' (e.g. Caron et al. 2013; Sanderson et al. 2017). This term sug-gests that one of the features that marks out this area of research is the relative fluidity of diagnosis. Although consensus statements position concussion as a parti-cularly difficult and complex condition to diagnose, athletes believe that they can diagnose concussion in both themselves and their team mates. We explore the changing role of lay medical knowledge in Chapter 8.

Second, and related to this self-definitional element, it is notable that there is no comparable body of research for other types of sporting injuries. While concussion research can be located in the broader literatures on pain and injury, and the social organization of sports medicine (Malcolm and Safai 2012), there is no other type of sporting injury for which researchers have sought to quantify how frequently ath-letes *do not* report their injuries. What we therefore see is that concussion research is in part driven by the *a priori* acceptance that concussion represents a distinct type of injury and therefore it is legitimate to subject it to distinct types of enquiry. This, in turn, serves to reinforce perceptions of the distinctiveness of concussion in the scientific and public imagination. The claims that concussions are chronically underreported are bereft of context and comparisons to give them meaning. More significantly, perhaps, the assumptions that lie behind this research reflect a crisis that is self-fuelling. The particular concerns of concussion serve to generate research which is almost predestined to enhance those concerns (i.e. the non-reporting of injury).

Third, consider the subjects of this body of research. Team sports involving physical contact predominate. Relatively absent are studies of participants in combat sports such as boxing and martial arts, despite the fact that the potential for longer-term neurocognitive decline was identified so much earlier. Additionally, a great deal of evidence on which we develop our understanding relates to younger sport participants. This may be the population for which fears of developing Chronic Traumatic Encephalopathy (CTE) are particularly emotive, but they are also the population for which evidence of a correlation between playing sport and developing longer-term neurocognitive conditions is the weakest. The condition of former players in the NFL first raises concerns about CTE as an 'occupational disease' and, if proven, there is a long way to go before it can be established that CTE is linked to less prolonged or intense engagement with football activities. There is then a clear ethical, medical, and cultural bias in this field towards certain populations.

These themes – medical knowledge, the 'uniqueness' of concussion, and youth focus – will form key parts of the analysis in Chapter 8. First, however, we look at the public health interventions that have been made as a consequence of the findings presented by the behavioural sciences, and the desire to resolve sport's concussion crisis.

Note

1 www.rugbyplayers.org/international-survey-highlights-player-concerns/

References

Anderson, L. and Jackson, S. (2012) 'Competing loyalties in sports medicine: threats to medical professionalism in elite commercial sport', *International Review of the Sociology of Sport*, 48(2): 238–256.

Bennett, L., Arias, J., Ford, P., Bernick, C., and Banks, S. (2018) 'Concussion reporting and perceived knowledge of professional fighters', *The Physician and Sports Medicine*, doi:10.1080/00913847.2018.1552481

Bloom, G.Horton, A., Johnston, K., and McCrory, P. (2004) 'Sport psychology and concussion: new impacts to explore', *British Journal of Sports Medicine*, 38: 519–521.

Broglio, S., Vagnozzi, R., Sabin, M., Signoretti, S., Tavazzi, B., and Lazzarino, G. (2010) 'Concussion occurrence and knowledge in Italian football (soccer)', *Journal of Sports Science and Medicine*, 9: 418–430.

Caron, J., Bloom, G., Johnston, K., and Sabiston, C. (2013) 'Effects of multiple concussion on retired National Hockey League players', *Journal of Sport & Exercise Psychology*, 35: 168–179.

Chinn, N. and Porter, P. (2016) 'Concussion reporting behaviours of community college student-athletes and limits of transferring concussion knowledge during the stress of competition', *BMJ Open Sport & Exercise Medicine*, 2: e000118.

Colón, A., Smith, S., and Fucillo, J. (2017) 'Concussions and risk within cultural contexts of play', *Qualitative Health Research*, 27(7): 1077–1089.

Delaney, J., Lacroix, V., Leclerc, S., and Johnston, K. (2002) 'Concussions among university football and soccer players', *Clinical Journal of Sport Medicine*, 12(6): 331–338.

Delaney, J., Lamfookon, C., Bloom, G., Al-Kashmiri, A., and Correa, J. (2015) 'Why university athletes choose not to reveal their concussion symptoms during a practice or game', *Clinical Journal of Sport Medicine*, 25(2): 113–125.

Fox, R.C. (2000) 'Medical uncertainty revisited', in G.L. Albrecht, R. Fitzpatrick, and S.C. Scrimshaw (eds.), *The Handbook of Social Studies in Health and Medicine*. London: SAGE, 409–425.

Fraas, M., Coughlan, G., Hart, E., and McCarthy, C. (2013) 'Concussion history and reporting rates in elite Irish rugby union players', *Physical Therapy in Sport*, 15(3):136–142.

Freidson, E. (1970) *Profession of Medicine: A Study of the Sociology of Applied Knowledge*. New York: Dodd, Mead & Co.

Hughes, R. and Coakley, J. (1991) 'Positive deviance among athletes: the implications of overconformity to the sport ethic', *Sociology of Sport Journal*, 8: 307–325.

Kerr, Z., Register-Mihalik, J., Kay, M., DeFreese, J.D., Marshall, S.W., and Gusiewicz, K. (2018) 'Concussion nondisclosure during professional career among a cohort of former National Football League athletes', *The American Journal of Sports Medicine*, 46(1): 22–29.

Kotarba, J. (2012) 'Women professional athletes' injury care: the case of women's football', in D. Malcolm and P. Safai (eds.), *The Social Organization of Sports Medicine: Critical Sociocultural Perspectives*. New York: Routledge, 107–125.

Kroshus, E., Baugh, C., Daneshvar, D., and Viswanath, K. (2014) 'Understanding concussion reporting using a model based on the theory of planned behavior', *Journal of Adolescent Health*, 54: 269–274.

Kroshus, E., Chrisman, S., Milroy, J., and Baugh, C. (2018) 'History of concussion diagnosis, differences in concussion reporting behaviour, and self-described reasons for non-report', *Journal of Clinical Sport Psychology*, doi:10.1123/jcsp.2017-0036

Kroshus, E., Garnett, B., Hawrilenko, M., and Baugh, C. (2015) 'Concussion under-reporting and pressure from coaches, teammates, fans and parents', *Social Science and Medicine*, 134: 66–75.

Liston, K., McDowell, M., Malcolm, D., Scott, A., and Waddington, I. (2018) 'On being "head strong": the pain zone and concussion in Non-Elite Rugby Union', *International Review for the Sociology of Sport*, 53(6): 668–684.

Malcolm, D. (2006) 'Unprofessional practice? The status and power of sports physicians', *Sociology of Sport Journal*, 23(4): 376–395.

Malcolm, D. (2009) 'Medical uncertainty and clinician-athlete relations: the management of concussion injuries in rugby union', *Sociology of Sport Journal*, 26(2): 191–210.

Malcolm, D. (2017) *Sport, Medicine and Health: The Medicalization of Sport?* London: Routledge.

Malcolm, D. (2018) 'Concussion in sport: public, professional and critical sociologies', *Sociology of Sport Journal*, 35(2): 141–148.

Malcolm, D. and Safai, P. (2012) *The Social Organization of Sports Medicine: Critical Socio-Cultural Perspectives*. New York: Routledge.

Malcolm, D. and Sheard, K. (2002) '"Pain in the assets": the effects of commercialization and professionalization on the management of injury in English Rugby Union', *Sociology of Sport Journal*, 19(2): 149–169.

Mathieu, F., Ellis, M., and Tator, C. (2018) 'Concussion education in Canadian medical schools: a 5 year follow-up survey', *BMC Medical Education*, 18: 316.

Messner, M. (1992) *Power at Play: Sport and the Problems of Masculinity*. Boston, MA: Beacon Press.

Mrazik, M., Dennison, C., Brooks, B., Yeates, K.O., Babul, S., and Naidu, D. (2015) 'A qualitative review of sports concussion education: prime time for evidence-based knowledge translation', *British Journal of Sports Medicine*, 49: 1548–1553.

Nixon, H.L. II (1992) 'A social network analysis of influences on athletes to play with pain and injuries', *Journal of Sport and Social Issues*, 16: 127–135.

O'Connell, E. and Molloy, M. (2016) 'Concussion in rugby: knowledge and attitudes of players', *Irish Journal of Medical Science*, 185: 521–528

Price, J., Malliaras, P., and Hudson, Z. (2012) 'Current practices in determining return to play following head injury in professional football in the UK', *British Journal of Sports Medicine*, 46: 1000–1003.

Register-Mihalik, J., Guskiewicz, K., Valovich McLeod, T., Linnan, L., Mueller, F., and Marshall, S. (2013) 'Knowledge, attitude, and concussion-reporting behaviors among high school athletes: a preliminary study', *Journal of Athletic Training*, 48(5): 645–653.

Roderick, M., Waddington, I., and Parker, G. (2000) 'Playing hurt: managing injuries in English professional football', *International Review for the Sociology of Sport*, 35: 165–180

Rosenbaum, A. and Arnett, P. (2010) 'The development of a survey to examine knowledge about and attitudes toward concussion in high-school students', *Journal of Clinical and Experimental Neuropsychology*, 32(1): 44–55.

Safai, P. (2003) 'Healing the body in the "culture of risk": examining the negotiations of treatment between sport medicine clinicians and injured athletes in Canadian inter-collegiate sport', *Sociology of Sport Journal*, 20(2): 127–146.

Sanderson, J., Weathers, M., Snedaker, K., and Gramlich, K. (2017) '"I was able to still do my job on the field and keep playing": an investigation of female and male athletes experiences with (not) reporting concussions', *Communication and Sport*, 5(3): 267–287.

Scott, A. (2012) 'Sport and exercise medicine's professional project: the impact of formal qualifications on the organization of British Olympic medical services', *International Review for the Sociology of Sport*, 49(5): 575–591.

Sye, G., Sullivan, J., and McCrory, P. (2006) 'High school rugby players' understanding of concussion and return to play guidelines', *British Journal of Sports Medicine*, 40: 1003–1005.

Theberge, N. (2007) '"It's not about health, it's about performance": sport medicine, health and the culture of risk in Canadian sport', in J. Hargreaves and P. Vertinsky (eds.), *Physical Culture, Power and the Body*. London: Routledge, 176–194.

Waddington, I. (2000) *Sport, Health and Drugs: A Critical Sociological Perspective*. London: E&FN Spon.

Walk, S. (1997) 'Peers in pain: the experiences of student athletic trainers', *Sociology of Sport Journal*, 14(1): 22–56.

Williams, J.M., Langdon, J.L., McMillan, J.L., and Buckley, T.A. (2016). 'English professional football players concussion knowledge and attitude', *Journal of Sport Health Science*, 5 (2): 197–204.

Wing, K., Bailey, H., Gronek, P., Podstawski, R., and Clark, C. (2018) 'A preliminary audit of medical and aid provision in English rugby union clubs: compliance with Regulation 9', *Irish Journal of Medical Science*, doi:10.1008/s11845–11018–1913-z

Young, K., and White, P. (1993). 'Sport, physical danger and injury: the experiences of elite women athletes', *Journal of Sport & Social Issues*, 19: 45–61.

7

CONCUSSION AND PUBLIC HEALTH

Ash read the leaflet. Of course head injuries were serious. Nobody disagreed with that. But it was one thing to read it in the changing room; another when you were on the pitch. While these people needed her, those people didn't understand. 'We can't let them destroy our sport'.

If the previous chapter highlighted how the behaviour of sport's 'insiders' contrasts with the 'external' public concerns about concussion, this chapter centres on the point at which these two worlds meet: public health. As noted in Chapter 3, a central response to sport's concussion crisis has been the introduction of a range of awareness campaigns. There are important geographical differences in these campaigns; ranging from presidential endorsement by Barack Obama and mandatory forms of educational provision in the US to campaigns in Europe, South Africa, Australia, and New Zealand which sports governing bodies have voluntarily instigated. There are, further, individuals and pressure groups seeking to persuade sports governing bodies to invoke even more precautionary actions. Indicative of how significant public health has become in this context, Concussion in Sport Group (CISG) consensus statements position education as an increasingly important aspect of the field (McCrory et al. 2009). The aim of this chapter, therefore, is to examine the development of these public health interventions: what impact have they had on sport's concussion crisis?

Public health interventions date from around the mid-nineteenth century. Through a combination of urbanization and industrialization, and the development of modern biomedical science, it became increasingly understood that (ill) health was not simply a consequence of fate or 'God's Will', but frequently stemmed from environmental conditions. Over time, public health campaigns have shifted from simply seeking to *educate* populations to more proactive forms of health *promotion*. The latest phase has been dubbed the New Public Health (Lupton 1995) to depict trends towards increasingly holistic approaches to behavioural change targeted at entire rather than discrete populations. Critics of these programmes have questioned whether the level of intervention into the lives of the target population can be justified, whether these programmes deliver what they promise, and the degree to which the potential unintended consequences may result in net negative effects on individual health (Nettleton and Bunton 1995).

As we will see, concussion campaigns are consistent with these broader social developments in public health. Equally, many of the more generic critiques of public health resonate with these concussion-specific campaigns. Thus, in this chapter we first explore the effectiveness of various educational programmes and the attempts made to develop more sophisticated theoretical and methodological strategies. Do these programmes work? If not, why not? We then look at an ongoing public campaign that has sought to put increasing pressure on rugby's governing bodies to reduce the incidence of both injury and concussion. What does this tell us about broader public debates about concussion?

Addressing the knowledge 'deficit'

As we saw in Chapter 6, while concerns about the 'underreporting' of concussions can best be understood through more cultural and multicausal explanatory models of behaviour, the belief that improving knowledge and awareness is fundamental to any solution remains central. Thus, Cusimano et al. (2009: 318) concluded that their study demonstrated 'serious deficiencies' in the concussion knowledge of participants, parents and coaches in Canadian minor hockey. While they highlighted the role of the media and marketing campaigns in creating learned behaviours and expectations that promoted injury tolerance (effectively the 'sport cultural norms' discussed in Chapter 6), and called for a shift in attitudes away 'from a focus on winning at all costs to one that encompasses health in all its dimensions' (Cusimano et al. 2009: 318), they endorsed programmes like Smart-Hockey as having the potential to abate the phenomenon of athletes simply disregarding concussion injuries.

Similar optimism was expressed at the early implementation phases of rugby union educational campaigns. When a study of New Zealand high school students found that less than half had seen, or been told about, concussion guidelines, and just 22 per cent had sought medical clearance to resume playing after a concussion, the authors concluded that the sample had 'at least a fundamental understanding of what constitutes concussion' (Sye et al. 2006: 1004). Sye et al. (2006: 1004) argued that, with national initiatives to more systematically educate coaches and medical staff already coming on stream, 'it can be *assumed* that this information is now being more extensively transmitted to the players' (emphasis added).

Showing the geographical diversity within sport's concussion crisis, a decade later O'Connell and Molloy (2016: 527) similarly concluded that a cohort of Irish adult rugby players surveyed prior to the introduction of any formal educational campaign 'possessed a relatively good knowledge level'. However, most expressed little concern about the potential dangers of concussion, would likely continue playing regardless of receiving a head injury, and identified their teammates and coaches as their primary sources of information about concussion symptoms and management. Alongside this optimistic assessment, O'Connell and Molloy (2016) encouraged the formal implementation of concussion awareness programmes.

Such faith in the value of introducing educational programmes now appears misplaced. While the governing bodies of major rugby playing nations have rolled out concussion awareness campaigns, a systematic review published in 2016 concluded that 'there is little evidence to support the effectiveness of such programmes' (Fraas and Burchiel 2016: 1212). In part, the lack of evidence is a consequence of only limited monitoring and evaluation but this, in itself, is indicative of a misplaced confidence that provision equates to behavioural change. Indeed, Fraas and Burchiel (2016) found that only ten evaluation studies had been conducted across the sport and only two rugby programmes – the *RugbySmart* programme in New Zealand and *BokSmart* in South Africa[1] – conformed to what has been outlined as good practice for the introduction of injury prevention models (based on baseline research, implementation and effectiveness monitoring). Fraas and Burchiel (2016) ultimately conclude that the only evidence for the effectiveness of these programmes is derived from poor quality sources (i.e. opinion- or case-study based), while good quality sources of data only provide evidence of general rather than concussion-specific effectiveness. More particularly, a review of Boksmart indicated that high-risk tackling and scrummaging behaviours had been reduced but provided no indication of the impact of this on concussion incidence. Similarly, it was found that RugbySmart had improved playing techniques and reduced foul play, improved injury prevention knowledge, and positively affected media messages about injury management. Crucially, however, Accident Compensation Corporation data reported in the New Zealand media suggest that *concussion injuries* were increasing in frequency.

Assessments of the CDC's Heads Up programme draw broadly similar conclusions. This campaign includes a range of different materials (booklets, videos, posters, factsheets, etc.) aimed at a variety of target audiences (e.g. high school, youth sport). Initially an evaluation of the impact of these resources on coaches suggested that knowledge, attitudes, and behaviour developed in line with the programme goals. For instance, 90 per cent of coaches reported using the resources, 82 per cent found them 'extremely useful', and 38 per cent reported changing their behaviours as a consequence (Sarmiento et al. 2010: 117). However, a subsequent study found that the education of coaches had minimal impact on their overall awareness of the incidence of concussion amongst their athletes (Rivara et al. 2014). Moreover, a study of the toolkit provided to physicians found that while a mailing intervention did result in a reduced likelihood of next-day return to play (RTP) (as recommended), it 'did not affect general concussion knowledge or response to concussion scenarios' (Chrisman et al. 2011: 1033). Once again, therefore, evidence gathering is limited and evidence for the effectiveness of the programmes that *have* been studied varies.

While it is clearly difficult to establish a cause-effect relationship between these social interventions and behavioural change (discussed later), part of the reason for such consistent programme failure must lie in implementation. Kroshus et al. (2014b) were among the first to point out that while concussion education had become mandatory across the US and enshrined in NCAA policy, nothing specific had been determined in terms of actual content or mode of delivery. Their subsequent research showed considerable variation in this regard, with some attending a lecture and others simply having handouts left 'for common perusal' (Kroshus et al. 2014b: 138). Consequently it could be argued that the mandate for the provision of material is necessary but not sufficient to invoke the desired change. Indeed, a later qualitative review of educational materials concluded that, at best, post-educational inventions with athletes showed evidence only of short-term improvements, while 'the long-term gains are mixed' (Mrazik et al. 2015: 1551).

Despite such muted qualitative gains, the quantitative growth of educational and awareness programmes has been significant. Mrazik et al. (2015) identified over 2000 journal articles focusing on sport/concussion, knowledge/education, and multiple webinars and online resources. Indeed, so buoyant is this market for concussion education that in addition to both sport and state funded free-to-access programmes, researchers found around 40 commercially provided applications available to download onto phones, tablets, etc.

Consequently, research has sought to examine the most effective media for dissemination with, again, mixed results. While some evidence exists that interactive resources are the most effective at improving understanding, others have argued that the use of video materials and quizzes is less effective than written materials or in-person training (Rivara et al. 2014). Ahmed et al. (2012) suggest that where social media are used to disseminate concussion information, moderation by a healthcare provider would ensure quality and accessibility and thus facilitate wider utilization. However, the proliferation of resources in this relatively unregulated market has had the unintended consequence of exposing athletes to the potential for economic exploitation through some commercially provided, yet factually questionable, educational programmes. That market becomes more lucrative as the concussion crisis continues.

There is also a clear concern that these developments could not only be failing to address, but actually *contributing to,* non-compliant behaviour. The potential *negative effect* of educational materials was illustrated through a comparison of three concussion awareness materials: the NATA and National Academy of Neuropsychology's *Concussion in Ice Hockey* video; the CDC's Heads Up factsheet; and the film/documentary *Head Games.* Across the sample, underreporting appeared to *increase* leading the authors to report 'cause for pessimism' (Kroshus et al. 2015b: 157). Moreover, in relation to the *Concussion in Ice Hockey* video in particular, the researchers witnessed highly irreverent behaviour amongst the research subjects who became rowdy and cheered footage of athletes in big collisions incurring concussion injuries. Thus 'it is possible that when professional hockey players described their experiences with concussion . . . they in fact normalized playing through injury' (Kroshus et al. 2015b: 157). The authors further speculate that athletes may even be experiencing a degree of information fatigue, having now been exposed to such educational materials for a significant number of years.

In line with this consistent theme of programme ineffectiveness, further attempts have been made to identify the sectors of the population which have the weakest knowledge. While in both the UK and Canada it has been recognized that athletes' 'poor' knowledge of concussion is in part a manifestation of the broader populations' ignorance of head injuries (Weber and Edwards 2012; Cusimano et al. 2017), echoing a finding reported in Chapter 3, Cusimano et al. (2017) argue that the more limited knowledge exhibited by Canada's francophone population may be indicative of a lower level of concern within non-anglophone sporting communities. Level of education and relative affluence have also been shown to correlate with the understanding of concussion exhibited in biomedical consensus statements (Cusimano et al. 2017; Kurowski et al. 2014). Finally, although it has also been argued that older and more competitive players exhibit better knowledge (Cusimano et al. 2009), as do those occupying key social/community roles (e.g. coaches, doctors, etc.), equally it has been noted that this knowledge deficit extends to healthcare professionals. Thus, while Cusimano et al. (2017) call for the development of more targeted education programmes, they also believe that improving the knowledge of the most knowledgeable groups (healthcare professionals and coaches) would pay dividends in raising awareness amongst the general population. Yet such is the apparent resilience of existing attitudes, even an intimate experience of head injury (either personally or through a close friend) seems to have little influence on changing concussion-related knowledge.

Towards a more sophisticated approach to behavioural change

In light of such policy failure, calls have increasingly been made for more complex and theoretically informed intervention models. Indicatively, Kroshus et al. (2014b: 136) cited a systematic review that found that 'sports injury prevention research finds that only 11% of studies, and no concussion education programmes for athletes, explicitly include theory in programme design, implementation or evaluation'. To this end Kroshus (with various colleagues) has perhaps been the most proactive, drawing on both social norms theory (Kroshus et al. 2015c) and the theory of planned behaviour (Kroshus et al. 2014a; 2015a) to understand respondent behaviour and inform programme design. Their aim has been to develop 'population specific and theory-driven educational interventions' (Kroshus et al. 2015b: 158).

Equally proactive has been Provvidenza, a leading advocate of applying knowledge transfer principles to inform concussion awareness materials. Knowledge transfer (KT) focusses on 'finding creative and effective ways' (Provvidenza and Johnston 2009: i68) to deliver the right kind of information to the right people at the right time so that it subsequently informs behaviour. Building on a foundational set of five questions – Who is the target audience? What is the message being delivered? Who is delivering the message? How is the message transferred? What is the impact of the knowledge transfer? – Provvidenza and Johnston tailor specific strategies to different target groups. For instance, it is argued that physicians respond best to education outreach, interactive education, and reminder messages (but poorly to traditional didactic lectures or printed/passive materials); physiotherapists/athletic therapists respond best to problem-based learning and evidence-based practice; coaches are most receptive to forms of in-action and on-action reflection; and a 'multiple intelligences' approach may be most effective when dealing with the inevitably more diverse student-athlete population.[2] In this respect the use of e-learning, television, video gaming (Provvidenza and Johnston 2009), and social media (Provvidenza et al. 2013) is recommended for programmes aimed at young people. Moreover, peer support groups have been assessed as effective in facilitating recovery. Yet as Provvidenza et al. (2013: 338) state, while KT is increasingly being used in relation to concussion, the 'effectiveness and overall impact require further insight and investigation'. Despite a lack of proven effectiveness, the latest CISG statement (McCrory et al. 2017) advocates the international development of concussion-related KT programmes.

Perhaps the central reason why these interventions have not signalled more dramatic behavioural changes is because they essentially remain rooted in the same key assumptions. For example, although KT recognizes co-existing forms of knowledge, it is premised on the belief that biomedically derived knowledge is and should be ascendant. While the explicit goals of KT appear to be relatively democratic – described for instance as multidirectional, interactive, non-linear, ongoing, interdisciplinary, impact oriented, involving multiple activities and multiple user groups but always in a user- and context-specific way (Provvidenza et al. 2013) – in practice, the concept of knowledge *transfer* will likely lead to other (lay) forms of knowledge being supplanted. While the increasing public and patient involvement in the formulation of health interventions is a more general trend in healthcare, existing research highlights the way in which medicine tends to do this on its own terms rather than genuinely seeking out and being shaped by alternative perspectives (Martin and Finn 2011).

A second problematic assumption is evident in the dominance of positivist approaches. Evaluation is invariably quantitative rather than qualitative (Mrazik et al. 2015), indicated in the continuing belief that evaluation needs 'controlled research studies' (Provvidenza and Johnson 2009: i74). While the evaluation of health promotion frequently tries to quantify essentially qualitative phenomena, here in particular it should be noted that as 'the objective means to measure concussive injury have not been established' (Cusimano et al. 2009: 315) attempts to objectively measure concussion-related behaviour are inherently flawed.

Third, and related to this, is the propensity to reductively treat complex behavioural patterns through isolating risk variables (e.g. identifying what percentage of respondents did not know they were concussed, or thought it was sufficiently serious to report, etc.). While these evaluations thus replicate a problem identifiable across public health interventions, it is on this basis that it is assumed that target audiences will ultimately act in line with the rationality of the implemented programme, and thus that developing knowledge will (eventually) lead to the behavioural change expected (a questionable assumption on the basis of the studies reviewed here). Tellingly, no educational campaigns have sought to address the phenomenon of risk compensation which essentially disrupts health rationality assumptions and which, since 2004, CISG statements have suggested may contribute to concussion incidence (see Chapter 4).

A fourth and additional issue is a lack of reflexivity on the limited nature of the biomedical understanding of concussion. There appears to be a misplaced conviction amongst biomedical scientists which blinds them to their fundamentally limited understanding of concussion and the scope this allows for alternative ways of viewing concussion to exist. The proposed solutions essentially focus on individual rather than cultural behavioural change, and in this respect they replicate the general psychologization of health promotion (Horrocks and Johnson 2014). An exception to this pattern is Kroshus et al. (2015b) who sought to test video delivered educational materials (as prior research had shown that this is what players thought would work) and suggest that the population may be more receptive to function-specific concussion advice, for example, emphasizing how reaction times slowed post-concussion. Overall it is rare that such research centrally sees human behaviour as socially determined. Moreover, as Gibson (2018) more generally notes, the voices of children and young people are largely absent in the debates over concussion; adults are effectively imposing ideas upon them.

Finally, as KT programmes show, there is a concern that different elements of the target community are differentially receptive to these programmes. Indeed, more generally, those who do respond as desired are those who already practice relatively safe and healthy behaviours (Baum and Fisher 2014). The outcome is the potential for interventions to ultimately *create* greater divisions between different sections of the community. Until it is demonstrated otherwise, therefore, there is the potential that concussion awareness programmes could lead to the polarization of behaviours. Thus, in many ways, concussion education programmes effectively replicate the problems identified in public health more generally and so may merely compound, rather than resolve, sport's concussion crisis.

Shaping the concussion public health debate

Partly in response to the lack of effectiveness of existing public health interventions, but equally because a more fundamental change is desired, some have embarked on campaigns to alter the existing structures of sport and, in particular, encourage the implementation of further and more radical rule changes. Perhaps the most notable individual in this regard has been Allyson Pollock. Pollock is co-author of a number of scientific studies (Kirkwood et al. 2015; Pollock et al. 2017) and opinion or advocacy pieces (Pollock and Kirkwood 2016; 2017) charting the incidence of injury in rugby union and the 'need' for change, has authored a book aimed at a public audience – *Tackling Rugby: What Every Parent Should Know* (Pollock 2014) – and co-founded a group called the Sport Collision Injury Collective (SCIC).

The centrepiece of the SCIC campaign has been an open letter – 'Preventing injuries in children playing school rugby' – sent in March 2016 to Children's Commissioners, Chief Medical Officers (CMOs) and Secretaries of State for Education, Health and Culture across the UK.[3] The letter argued that rugby entails a high rate of often serious injury; that it was a compulsory part of the PE curriculum in many UK secondary schools (11–16 years); that the majority of injuries stem from contact or collision; that head injury and concussion are common and potentially more problematic for children; and that rugby injuries result in children's significant time loss from school and reduced participation in the game. In conclusion, the letter recommended a ban on contact in school-based rugby union in the UK and Ireland. As befitting this cultural crisis, the campaign attracted considerable global media attention and was debated within sports medicine journals. An analysis of both the public and academic debates surrounding this campaign not only develops our discussion of concussion and public health, but sheds light on the way such debates are performed and helps us to understand more about the divided opinions that underpin sport's concussion crisis.

While it is difficult to assess the overall balance of public approval/dispute with the campaign, clearly evident was some formalized and co-ordinated resistance to the campaign which came from four primary sources. First, the Association for Physical Education (AfPE) published a statement giving 'full' support to the inclusion of rugby in the National Curriculum for PE (NCPE) and expressed being 'extremely frustrated and disappointed at the claims made . . . [which represent] an attack on the skills' of those who taught rugby in schools.[4] A blog written by an academic and former PE teacher, and published by the *British Journal of Sports Medicine*, was further critical of the campaign. Gibson (2018) argued that the unqualified citations 'of "compulsory rugby" in schools are unhelpfully vague, potentially disingenuous and antagonistic and as such have stymied meaningful debate'. It was further argued that the extrapolation of existing injury data to ~ies incurred in physical education was problematic due to the significant con~ differences. Gibson (2018) concluded by echoing the AfPE position ~ the professionalism of PE teachers, arguing that the current UK cur~ ~wers educators to teach activities that best reflect their expertise, ~ds of their students'.

~mbers of the medical community argued that restrictions on ~ be resisted due to the potential for a negative net effect ~r three US paediatricians – MacDonald and Myer ~(2017) – concern about sedentary behaviours was ~ the risks posed by head injuries to youth popu~ ~personnel expressed similar concerns. As Calder~ ~'although not everyone can win Olympic gold, ~ . . . these [are] unquestioned benefits . . . [the ~itant danger of causing disengagement with sport, ~l'. Bullingham et al. (2017: 1450) responded by ~r had not called for 'the banning of sports, or for children to become sedentary, nor is it targeted at the structure of community rugby where parents and children opt voluntarily to participate'.

Third, some members of what might be called the rugby community reacted with a robust defence. Former England player Will Greenwood passionately issued the following response, aired on the UK's major sports broadcaster *Sky TV*. Greenwood stated:

> You can keep your stats and your numbers because it is what a sport gives you – that feeling of being together as one and of building something.
>
> [It] gives the values we hold dear in sport: respect, team-ship, the ability to stand side by side. To me that is far more important than the occasional niggle and the occasional scrape.
>
> I am passionate in believing that we have a cotton wool nanny state that continually tells me what I can and cannot do. Life is about taking knocks and then getting back up off the floor and going again, and going again, and going again.
>
> I understand your values but are you telling me right now that you want rugby banned? I have never ever heard such nonsense in my entire life.[5]

What can only be partially portrayed through this text is Greenwood's heightened emotion – though indicative of this, perhaps, is his misreading of the campaign (there was no attempt to ban rugby). This 'misreading' is actually very revealing for it shows how he links the game to such fundamental issues as identity and personal character and interprets proposals for change as either an existential or axiological threat. But Greenwood's response is worth quoting at length because it also illustrates a number of salient features of the wider debate. In this extract we can see: the contestation of different forms of evidence; the misrepresentation of opponents; a defence of the status-quo; commitment to the sport-health ideology; refusal to compromise; and ultimately the suggestion that this movement is part of a larger, pernicious social movement (the 'cotton wool nanny state'). It was clear from this, and indeed some even more vociferous responses and personal attacks, just how deep the divisions are within sport's concussion crisis.

Fourth, and most decisively, the CMOs rejected the SCIC's conclusion and recommendations, claiming that they were unsupported by the evidence. response illustrates some of the issues previously raised, it the mobilization of 'facts' to support data and the nat debate. The response was directly informed by th CMOs Physical Activity Expert Group (PAEG). had previously been assembled to provide advice activity (rather than sport per se). While the com claim that the group 'has a wide membership of teacher education, emergency care, sports science loskeletal medicine], paediatrics, epidemiology, performance/elite sports medicine', the reality i

natural science bias with little if any expertise in matters relating to *school sport*. [6]
Rather the membership shows the hallmarks of a group assembled to provide expert
advice about the health benefits of physical activity, rather than a more holistic view
of sport and its potential dangers. No additional physical education, ethics, sports
injury, or concussion expertise was seconded to augment the group. Why then was
this group deemed to have either the necessary or desirable expertise to respond to
the issues raised? The deployment of the PAEG suggests that the CMOs primarily
understood these issues through their pre-existing commitment to the sport-health
ideology. It further indicates a (misplaced) faith on the ability of biomedical science
to resolve social and ethical issues. Ultimately, it raises questions about the openness
of the CMOs to a debate over the negative health consequences of sports and related
exercise activities (see Chapter 8).

The *detail* of the response provided by the PAEG led Piggin and Bairner (2019)
to ask 'what counts as "the evidence"?' The PAEG disputed that rugby was a
compulsory part of PE; a claim that is reasonable in that the NCPE does not
demand the playing of rugby, but *misleading* in that the NCPE does allow individual
schools to set a PE curriculum in which rugby is compulsory (Gibson 2018). The
PAEG also countered the SCIC's claim that concussion was a common injury by
suggesting that increased education and awareness meant 'that it may be now that
true concussion is over-reported, making it currently difficult to ascertain where the
true incidence lies' (emphasis added). This statement was not supported by any evidence and, in light of the earlier discussion of epidemiology (see Chapter 4),
appears at odds with the more broadly established biomedical position on the
incidence of concussion. Perhaps most damningly, however, Piggin and Bairner
(2019) argued that the PAEG constructed a 'straw-person' argument (a criticism
that could also be raised at Will Greenwood). In stating that 'not allowing children
to play or be active will be detrimental to their emotional, social, mental and
physical health', they inferred that the SCIC campaign was anti-physical activity
per se (the topic on which the committee had essentially been assembled to advise
upon in the first place and thus a position they were inevitably going to oppose).
The PAEG criticized the SCIC for not listing 'the educational, health, social or
mental benefits of participation and as a result is selective in its reporting of data',
yet concluded that 'we think the benefits of experiencing, learning, training and
playing rugby, with appropriate supervision, safety and coaching, considerably
outweigh the risks of injury'. Ironically this statement was made without: 1) providing any evidence of those benefits; 2) undertaking any assessment of whether
existing supervision, safety and coaching in schools was 'appropriate'; and 3)
explicitly claiming that the 'true incidence' of rugby injuries 'remains contentious'.
Evidently the opposing sides of the concussion crisis are frequently talking past,
rather than to, each other (see Chapter 9).

The campaign has also brought into sharper focus some of the claims made by
rugby governing bodies and, in particular, the way the risks associated with playing
the sport are portrayed. While the IRB had explicitly accepted that 'a risk is associated with head injury and concussion even if this risk is unquantifiable and

unknown' (cited in Partridge and Hall, 2014: 42), the CEO of *World Rugby* was compelled to issue an apology and retraction after Piggin and Pollock (2017) published a critique of the 'erroneous and misleading' representation of Australian sports injury statistics. It was argued that World Rugby had replicated the common fallacy of conflating sport (specifically rugby) and exercise or physical activity, and unproblematically transposed the well-rehearsed health benefits of the latter onto the former (see the discussion of the sport-health ideology in Chapter 8). World Rugby were further critiqued for failing to substantiate their claim that a survey had found that 'most parents say the benefits of sport outweighs (sic) the risks' (Piggin and Pollock 2017: 1108). Indeed, it was noted that an important feature of this information was not simply that it was incorrect, but that the data sources consistently showed the *opposite* of what World Rugby claimed for them. Piggin (2017; Piggin and Bairner 2017) subsequently critiqued the 'misleading official claims' published in *England Rugby*'s 'Rugby Safe' booklet and called for an immediate end to 'the obfuscation of actual injury rates by rugby organisations'. England Rugby (a rebranding of the RFU) withdrew the booklet and apologized for the errors it contained, clearly recognizing their duty to sufficiently represents the risk of the activities they regulate (see Chapter 5).[7]

A further response to the SCIC campaign was published by Quarrie et al. (2017). They positioned the debate as essentially a clash of values between a group who saw childhood injuries as 'inherently undesirable' and those that viewed injuries as an 'acceptable compromise' given the potential benefits of participation (Quarrie et al. 2017: 1134). They further argued that injury rates were a question of fact that could be quantified (as we have seen, a somewhat problematic statement) but rightly emphasized that: 1) risk had to be viewed relationally as either *relatively* high or low; and 2) that the evaluation of risk will always be 'value dependent'. Indicatively they cited Starr's (1969) estimate that where risks are voluntary, people's acceptable levels were roughly 1000 times higher than where the activity/risks are involuntary. Echoing the ethical discussion cited earlier (see Chapter 5), they note that regulation needs to be balanced against issues of liberty and personal autonomy and, in relation to this, the debate evident in sport's concussion crisis should be located within a wider social clash of values about the acceptability of risk to young people within the injury prevention community (a point developed in Chapter 8). While clear that our current knowledge of risk in incomplete, Quarrie et al. (2017: 1134) conclude that the risks of playing rugby 'do not appear to be inordinately high compared with a range of other childhood sports and activities'.

Conclusion

We can see that concussion-related public health interventions are largely failing to change sport participants' behaviour. This may be due to weakness in design, implementation, or more fundamentally perhaps due to broader conceptual issues. In this, concussion awareness educational programmes are not exceptional and indeed resonate with a number of sociological critiques of public health more generally. While 'finding a balance between advocacy and science is an ongoing challenge for those who work in health promotion and injury prevention' (Quarrie et al. 2017: 1138), a more fundamental issue may be the deployment of a model that fails to understand and directly address the values, concerns, and ideologies of sport participants. As the discussion of these broader debates shows, educational campaigns simply appear to be failing to reach out to the groups whose behaviour they are seeking to change. Quarrie et al. (2017) are surely correct to state that any solution must represent the values of a 'specific community' but ultimately this raises the question of who would actually constitute the community, for as we have seen, a cultural crisis involves a spill-over incorporating diverse groups and deep social divisions. In the next chapter, therefore, we explore the basis of these divisions: what kind of society is it in which this kind of crisis over concussion in sport has developed?

Notes

1 The two programmes have slightly different emphases. *RugbySmart* requires all coaches and referees to attend annual educational sessions which cover aspects such as physical conditioning, playing techniques, and injury management. *BokSmart* provides biennial compulsory workshops, online support materials, a telephone injury assistance hotline, and first aid training in deprived communities.
2 This approach is based on a belief that humans have seven discrete areas of intelligence, that individuals have specific strengths and weaknesses, and thus the most effective form of communication rests on identify which individuals will be most receptive to specific modalities of intelligence.
3 Details of the letter and the responses received can be found at www.sportcic.com/
4 www.afpe.org.uk/physical-education/afpe-statement-on-banning-tackling-in-school-rugby/ Accessed 27 September 2017.
5 www.skysports.com/rugby-union/news/12325/9172514/will-greenwood-reacts-to-the-suggestion-that-rugby-rules-need-to-be-changed Accessed 15 November 2018.
6 Group members were: Professor Charlie Foster (with research interests in public health and epidemiology); Dr Hamish Reid (with research interests in prehospital medicine); Dr George Bownes (sport and exercise medicine registrar); Stuart Fairclough (Professor of Physical Activity Education, with research interests in physical activity measurement and the role of multidimensional correlates in the promotion of physically active lifestyles among young people); Professor Gareth Stratton (specialising in paediatric exercise physiology); Dr Andrew Murray (with research interests in human physiology and sports medicine); Professor Melvyn Hillsdon (with research interests in epidemiology and public health); Dr Karen Milton (with research interests in sports science, public health and public policy); Professor Marie Murphy (with research interests in exercise physiology and biochemistry); Professor Nanette Mutrie (with research interests in exercise psychology); Dr Wilby Williamson (working in a cardiovascular clinical research facility).
7 https://physicalactivitypolitics.com/2017/07/20/an-urgent-call-for-clarity-regarding-england-rugbys-injury-claims-update/ Accessed 15 November 2018.

References

Ahmed, O., Sullivan, S., Schneiders, A. et al. (2012) 'iSupport: do social networking sites have a role to play in concussion awareness?', *Disability Rehabilitation*, 32: 1877–1883.

Baum, F. and Fisher, M. (2014) 'Why behavioural health promotion endures despite its failure to reduce health inequalities', *Sociology of Health and Illness*, 36(2): 213–225.

Bullingham, R., White, A., and Batten, J. (2017) 'Response to: "Don't let kids play football": a killer idea', *British Journal of Sports Medicine*, 51(20): 1450.

Calderwood, C., Murray, A., and Stewart, W. (2016) 'Turning people into couch potatoes is not the cure for sports concussion', *British Journal of Sports Medicine*, 50(4): 200–201.

Chrisman, S., Shiff, M., and Rivara, F. (2011) 'Physician concussion knowledge and the effect of mailing the CDC's "Heads Up" toolkit', *Clinical Pediatrics*, 50(11): 1031–1039.

Cusimano, M., Chipman, M.Volpe, R., and Donnelly, P. (2009) 'Canadian minor hockey participants' knowledge about concussion', *The Canadian Journal of Neurological Sciences*, 36: 315–320.

Cusimano, M., Zhang, S., Topolovec-Vranic, J., Hutchison, M., and Jing, R. (2017) 'Factors affecting the concussion knowledge of athletes, parents, coached and medical professionals', *SAGE Open Medicine*, 5: 1–9.

Fraas, M. and Burchiel, J. (2016) 'A systematic review of education programmes to prevent concussion in rugby union', *European Journal of Sport Science*, 16(8): 1212–1218.

Gibson, K. (2018) 'Banning the tackle in school rugby: let's put it into context', *British Journal of Sports Medicine Blog*, https://blogs.bmj.com/bjsm/2018/01/30/banning-tackle-school-rugby-lets-put-context/

Horrocks, C. and Johnson, S. (2014) 'A socially situated approach to inform health and wellbeing', *Sociology of Health and Illness*, 36(2): 175–186.

Kirkwood, G., Parekh, N., Ofori-Asenso, R., and Pollock, A.M. (2015) 'Concussion in youth rugby union and rugby league: a systematic review', *British Journal of Sports Medicine*, 49: 506–510.

Kroshus, E., Baugh, C., Daneshvar, D., and Viswanath, K. (2014a) 'Understanding concussion reporting using a model based on the theory of planned behavior', *Journal of Adolescent Health*, 54: 269–274.

Kroshus, E., Daneshvar, D., Baugh, C., Nowinski, C., and Cantu, R. (2014b) 'NCAA concussion education in ice hockey: an ineffective mandate', *British Journal of Sports Medicine*, 48: 135–140.

Kroshus, E., Garnett, B., Hawrilenko, M., and Baugh, C. (2015a) 'Concussion under-reporting and pressure from coaches, teammates, fans and parents', *Social Science and Medicine*, 134: 66–75.

Kroshus, E., Baugh, C., Hawrilenko, M., and Daneshvar, D. (2015b) 'Pilot randomized evaluation of publicly available concussion education materials: evidence of a possible negative effect', *Health Education and Behaviour*, 42(2): 153–162.

Kroshus, E., Garnett, B., Baugh, C., and Calzo, J. (2015c) 'Social norms theory and concussion education', *Health Education Research*, 30(6): 1004–1013.

Kurowski, B., Pemerantz, W., Schaiper, C. et al. (2014) 'Factors that influence concussion knowledge and self-reported attitudes in high school athlete', *Journal of Trauma Acute Care Surgery*, 77: S18–S22.

LaBella, C. and Myer, G. (2017) 'Youth sports injury prevention: keep calm and play on', *British Journal of Sports Medicine*, 51(3): 145–146.

Lupton, D. (1995) *The Imperative of Health. Public Health and the Regulated Body*. London: SAGE.

MacDonald, J. and Myer, G. (2017) '"Don't let kids play football": a killer idea', *British Journal of Sports Medicine*, 51(20): 1452–1453.

McCrory, P., Meeuwisse, W., Dvorak, J. et al. (2017) 'Consensus statement on concussion in sport: the 5th international conference on concussion in sport held in Berlin, October 2016', *British Journal of Sports Medicine*, 51: 838–847.

McCrory, P., Meeuwisse, W., Johnston, K. et al. (2009) 'Consensus statement on concussion in sport: the 3rd international conference on concussion in sport held in Zurich, November 2008', *British Journal of Sports Medicine*, 43(Suppl 1): i76–i80.

Martin, G. and Finn, R. (2011) 'Patients as team members: opportunities, challenges and paradoxes of including patients in multi-professional healthcare teams', *Sociology of Health and Illness*, 33(7): 1050–1065.

Mrazik, M., Dennison, C., Brooks, B., Yeates, K.O., Babul, S., and Naidu, D. (2015) 'A qualitative review of sports concussion education: prime time for evidence-based knowledge translation', *British Journal of Sports Medicine*, 49: 1548–1553.

Nettleton, S. and Bunton, R. (1995) 'Sociological critiques of health promotion', in R. Bunton, S. Nettleton and R. Burrows (eds.), *The Sociology of Health Promotion: Critical Analyses of Consumption, Lifestyle and Risk*, London: Routledge, 39–56.

O'Connell, E. and Molloy, M. (2016) 'Concussion in rugby: knowledge and attitudes of players', *Irish Journal of Medical Science*, 185: 521–528

Partridge, B. (2014) 'Dazed and confused: sports medicine, conflicts of interest, and concussion management', *Bioethical Inquiry*, 11: 65–74.

Piggin, J. (2017) 'Rugby, risk and rhetoric: the trivialisation of injury data must end', *New Zealand Journal of Sports Medicine*, 44(1): 8–9.

Piggin, J. and Bairner, A. (2017) 'An urgent call for clarity regarding England Rugby's injury claims', *Nordic Sport Science Forum*, http://idrottsforum.org/feature-piggin-bairner170523/

Piggin, J. and Bairner, A. (2019) 'What counts as 'the evidence'? A need for an urgent review of injury risk in school rugby', *British Journal of Sports Medicine*, 53: 10–11.

Piggin, J. and Pollock, A. (2017) 'World rugby's erroneous and misleading representation of Australian sports' injury statistics', *British Journal of Sports Medicine*, 51(15): 1108.

Pollock, A.M., White, A.J., and Kirkwood, G. (2017) 'Evidence in support of the call to ban the tackle and harmful contact in school rugby: a response to World Rugby', *British Journal of Sports Medicine*, 51: 1113–1117.

Pollock, A. (2014) *Tackling Rugby: What Every Parent Should Know about Injuries*. London: Verso.

Pollock, A. and Kirkwood, G. (2016) 'Removing contact from school rugby will not turn children into couch potatoes', *British Journal of Sports Medicine*, 50: 963–964.

Pollock, A. and Kirkwood, G. (2017) 'Tackle and scrum should be banned in school rugby', *British Medical Journal*, https://blogs.bmj.com/bmj/2017/09/25/allyson-pollock-and-graham-kirkwood-tackle-and-scrum-should-be-banned-in-school-rugby/

Provvidenza, C. and Johnson, K. (2009) 'Knowledge transfer principles as applied to sport concussion education', *British Journal of Sports Medicine*, 43(Suppl 1): i68–75.

Provvidenza, C., Engebretsen, L., Tator, C. et al. (2013) 'From consensus to action: knowledge transfer, education and influencing policy on sports concussion', *British Journal of Sports Medicine*, 47: 332–338.

Quarrie, K., Brookes, J., Burger, N., Hume, P., and Jackson, S. (2017) 'Facts and values: on the acceptability of risks in children's sport using the example of rugby: a narrative review', *British Journal of Sports Medicine*, 51: 1134–1139.

Rivara, F., Schiff, M., Chrisman, S., Chung, S., Ellenbogen, R., and Herring, S. (2014) 'The effect of coach education on reporting of concussions among high school athletes after passage of a concussion law', *The American Journal of Sports Medicine*, 42(5): 1197–1203.

Sarmiento, K., Mitchko, J., Klein, C., and Wong, S. (2010) 'Evaluation of the Centers for Disease Control and Prevention's concussion initiative for high school coaches: "Heads Up: Concussion in High School Sports"', *Journal of School Health*, 80(3): 112–118.

Starr, C. (1969) 'Social benefit versus technological risk', *Science*, 165: 1232–1238.

Sye, G., Sullivan, J. and McCrory, P. (2006) 'High school rugby players' understanding of concussion and return to play guidelines', *British Journal of Sports Medicine*, 40: 1003–1005.

Weber, M. and Edwards, M. (2012) 'Sport concussion knowledge in the UK general population', *Archives of Clinical Neuropsychology*, 27: 355–361.

8

THE SOCIAL ROOTS OF SPORT'S CONCUSSION CRISIS

There were some things Ash understood. Sport was fun. Sport makes you healthy. Doctors perform miracles. But there were some things she couldn't. Why was mum so over-protective? Why did Grandad keep forgetting her name? And how come those athletes on TV seem to play week after week? It all just seemed so complicated. 'How can we make sense of this?'

In 1950s and 1960s America, a debate arose about the growing number of young boys playing football and the related potential for injury. Bachynski (2019) highlights how such debates included reference to: the weakness of existing epidemiological knowledge; obfuscating comparative claims about which sports were the most dangerous; calls for the abolition of tackle football (for some age groups); a belief that appropriate adult supervision and instruction would be sufficient to remove potential harms; and *a priori* commitments to the value of participating in sport to enhance physical and mental health. Bachynski (2019: 2) further shows how public and medical concerns about the health risks of playing football 'were connected to broader cultural trends'. Of particular importance in this context were: the emerging professional interests of sports medicine; the Cold War, fears about the 'softening' of American youth, and the impact on national defence; and a commitment to the value of sport as a sphere in social life where individual masculinity and a collective sense of American patriotism could be developed. 'The conceptualization of football injuries as a medical issue was thus deeply tied up with ideological, moralistic, religious, and even nationalistic beliefs about the role of youth sports, as well as the country's direction more broadly' (Bachynski 2019: 24).

Through these historical events we can see elements of continuity and change. As debates about the risks of injury have reoccurred they have become entrenched upon similar value positions. But as noted at the beginning of Chapter 2, not all issues become social issues and not all social issues escalate into cultural crises.

Indeed, these earlier debates relatively quickly and peacefully dissipated. Thus, to explain the differences between these earlier concerns and the current concussion crisis, we need to examine the social context in which contemporary debates have occurred. Our task in this chapter, therefore, is to reveal the social roots of sport's concussion crisis.

Before embarking on that analysis, it is worth consolidating what we have established so far. We began by considering the concept of cultural crisis, the core features of which are not simply the existence of an important social problem that needs to be 'fixed', but a fundamental division between different communities. Subsequent chapters have detailed how the concussion crisis has come to 'spill-over' into more and more sports, various levels of competitiveness, and more geographically dispersed nations. Sports have revised their rules and medical regulations, embarked on research programmes, been subject to various political and legal interventions, and scrutinized by the cultural industries. Concussion has consequently come to attain a special cultural and medical status: not only a critical issue but uniquely regulated.

We subsequently explored the medical and ethical underpinnings to contemporary approaches to concussion. While concussion science has become formalized and more coherent in recent years, advances in knowledge relating to key features such as diagnosis, rehabilitation, incidence, and longer-term prognosis have been relatively few and far between. Consequently, concussion consensus statements take a rather contrary position, combining CTE-scepticism with an increasingly precautionary and paternalistic approach to SRC, particularly in relation to the regulation of youth sport. We subsequently (partly) explained this approach in relation to the peculiar ethical challenges of head injury and the distinct responsibilities assumed by sports governing bodies as dominant self-regulators.

Finally, we looked at research into the practices of sports participants and the public health interventions designed to reduce harm. These discussions showed that the existing and relatively precautionary forms of concussion regulation were both difficult to implement and widely rejected by the public at whom they were aimed. While currently implemented programmes could be improved, the broader debates invoked by campaigning groups shows just how deeply riven are the opposite sides of this cultural crisis.

The contemporary crisis is perhaps unique in that it: 1) is multisport and global in scope; 2) has entailed a more formalized and extensive medical investigation; and 3) has been subject to far-reaching yet unsuccessful attempts at behavioural change. But in seeking to understand the social roots of sport's concussion crisis, a wider range of factors must be considered. Here we draw upon the sociologies of health and medicine, childhood and ageing and, of course, sport. The aim is not to construct some kind of causal link between these social processes and sport's concussion crisis, but simply to connect concussion debates to broader social trends so that we can better understand this deep-rooted conflict. In the final chapter we consider future resolution, but first we ask: what kind of society is it in which concerns about sport-induced head injury come to assume such cultural significance?

Health and medicine

Previous sociological analyses have sought to understand debates surrounding SRC in relation to medicalization (Malcolm 2017; 2019). Briefly stated, medicalization describes the process whereby an increasing range of 'normal' everyday activities (e.g. sport) become subsumed into the medical domain. Medicalization occurs across three different areas: the conceptual, where a biomedical *perspective* come to structure public understanding of particular aspects of social life; the institutional, where biomedical *practices* are used to administer social problems; and the interactional, where biomedical *actors* become central to the 'cure' of social problems (Conrad 1992). On this basis we can, for example, see that the cultural fascination with CTE shows evidence of medicalization at the conceptual level; that institutional level medicalization includes the production of consensus statements, a standardized definition of concussion, the introduction of the SCAT and graduated return-to-play protocols, etc.; but that medicalization at the interactional level is the least developed, as the historical traditions and peculiar relations within the sport setting, create sources of resistance to medical control (see, e.g. the discussions of regulation in Chapter 4, the ethics of medical practice in Chapter 5, and responses to the clinical management of concussion in Chapter 6). While there remains a potential risk that the more SRC comes to be seen as a condition requiring medical management the more the lay population will become de-skilled (which could restrict the availability of concussion management 'expertise'), most evidence suggests that medical management is not replacing lay management of SRC but, ultimately, stepping into a vacuum. It is only in societies that have been extensively medicalized that sport's concussion crisis could emerge.

But while the medicalization of society has been broadly felt, it has not been without resistance. Following medical discoveries identifying a wider spectrum of conditions, and more subtle distinctions *within* known conditions, advances in medical treatment have continually been accompanied by uncertainty (Fox 2000). This has increased public awareness of the limited efficacy of medicine and a 'new medical pluralism' has developed, based on beliefs about the potential of complementary and alternative forms of medicine (Cant and Sharma 1999). These replace the paradigmatic reliance on randomized control trials to create evidence-based medicine with more holistic approaches which give greater emphasis to the social and emotional dimensions of disease (Gale 2011). Fuelled by neoliberal ideas about the role of consumer choice, and technological changes that allow patient communities to share and coordinate evidence, lay medical knowledge has become increasingly socially influential. This greater dependence on the embodied experience of illness is particularly apparent in the ideas discussed in Chapter 6, as: 1) we see considerable validity given to individuals' self-diagnosis of concussion; and 2) patients in elite sport exert a considerable influence over clinicians' understandings, diagnoses, and management of concussion. Social changes in the relationship between medicine and its patients are thus manifest in sport's concussion crisis.

Changes in the role of medicine within society have also led to a significant revision of the very idea of what it means to be 'healthy' which, again, is manifest in sport's concussion crisis. Shortly after World War II, the World Health Organization (WHO) published a definition of health which at the time was thought remarkably broad: 'a state of complete physical, mental and social well-being and not merely the absence of disease or infirmity' (cited in Huber et al. 2011). Just 60 years on, however, the control of contagious diseases, the corresponding growth in the relative significance of noncommunicable but chronic conditions, and an increasingly ageing population made this definition redundant. Complete well-being and absence of limitation are impractical and rarely achieved goals as huge numbers of people continually use various medications ranging, for example, from the use of over-the-counter paracetamol to intravenously administering insulin to control diabetes. In this context, it was proposed, health – physical, mental, and social – should be defined as 'the ability to adapt or self manage' (Huber et al. 2011: 1). Debates over SRC relate to this conception of health as self-management; there is a great experiential difference between those for whom the condition is a minor and temporary inconvenience and those for whom the continuous and uncontrollable nature of symptoms makes self-management challenging. Concussion straddles our contemporary understanding of (ill-)health and creates very different perceptions of the 'problem'.

This redefinition effectively consolidates existing cultural understandings of health. Crawford (1980), for instance, argued that health (in the West at least) had come to be understood as something that can and *must* be individually achieved (and hence Huber et al.'s emphasis on adaptation and self-management was already a social if not medical reality). But Crawford further argued that this meant that health had become incorporated into contemporary notions of character, identity, and citizenship such that those who failed to adopt healthy practices are deemed irresponsible, weak and personally culpable. The distinction between health and illness becomes increasingly blurred with the growth of preventative medicine and the increasing focus on the treatment of disease precursors through the life-course (Aronowitz 2009). It is in this context that public health interventions designed to enable people to recognize the signs and symptoms of concussion are seen as normal and valid, and that the non-compliant behaviour of sports populations is seen as a socially irresponsible choice to be 'corrected' using ever more sophisticated intervention models. The increasing medical focus on lifestyle underpins concerns about the connections between concussion and longer-term neurocognitive conditions such as ALS and CTE.

Consequently, people are increasingly expected to be 'autonomous, directed at self-improvement, self-regulated, desirous of self-knowledge' (Lupton 1995: 11). The 'civilized body' (Elias 2000) is increasingly able to exert a high degree of control over emotions, monitor the behaviour of others, and internalize ideas about appropriate/ desirable behaviour and body shape. Health, then, is not merely about self-management but reveals the more fundamental, internalized drive for self-control. It is in this context that health becomes increasingly intertwined, if not synonymous, with fitness (Glassner 1990; Bauman, 2000). People exercise to control/shape their bodies and the physical consequences of this 'work' are interpreted as an indication of good health/bodily self-management and control. We return to these issues in our later discussion of sport-related social changes, but for now it is important to note that what makes these ideas so pertinent to sport's concussion crisis is that the logical extrapolation of a holistic conception of health (physical, mental, social) which rests on the desire to rationalize the body (actions, emotions) leads us directly to the growing social prominence of brain health and neuroscience.

Brain Culture (Johnson Thornton 2011) entails a number of interacting processes that shape contemporary attitudes towards the brain. These include: the development of imaging techniques which render the living brain observable; the development of brain-related pharmaceuticals (the sale of psychiatric drugs in America increased by 600 per cent between 1990 and 2000); the growing market for brain training products (forecast to quadruple in value to $8.06bn between 2016 and 2021);[1] and the expansion of 'definitions of mental health and illness . . . to the point where virtually any aspect of life . . . can be located under the purview of mental health' (Johnson Thornton 2011: 132). Changing conceptualizations of health to embrace bodily self-control, therefore directly feed into changing social attitudes towards the brain.

As noted in Chapter 5, the brain has come to be seen as holding the essence of humanity; as fundamental to our consciousness, will, and emotions. The brain is viewed as what distinguishes humans as a species and people as individuals within that species. This facilitates the positioning of brain injuries as qualitatively distinct and distinctly more problematic than injury to any other part of the body. Equally, it facilitates our autonomy over health: if brains define human essence, then logically it follows that only 'I' properly understand my own brain. But brain health has also been repositioned in line with health in general; that is to say, as something that is malleable and therefore as something that we as individuals 'should' nurture and develop through lifestyle. Brain-based healthism opens up 'endless projects of self-optimization', and a cultural shift from 'you must be like this' to 'be all you can' (Johnson Thornton 2011: 2).

Sport's concussion crisis is inextricably tied to these developments. *Brain Culture* explains the historical shift from injury signalled by blood to injury signalled by cognitive failure (see Chapter 2). Just as brain norms are thought to be both diverse and personalized, so concussion affects people across such a wide range of symptoms and individual baseline testing is believed to enhance diagnosis. While SRC is a good example of the limitations of contemporary brain imaging techniques, and the current limited understanding of CTE is a salient reminder of medical uncertainty, growing concerns about managing head injuries flow from society's increasing confidence in, and expectations of, the efficacy of neuroscience. The case against the NFL, it will be remembered, was effectively premised on the belief that neuroscience would *at some point in the future* reveal a direct relationship between football participation and CTE. But seminal in changing attitudes towards mental health, Johnson Thornton (2011) argues, was President George W. Bush's comprehensive review of mental health care in the US first announced in April 2002. Mike Webster's death occurred just five months later and thus in the context of heightened political and media interest in mental health. This is surely one reason why Webster acted as a catalyst for sport's concussion crisis, why his death had so much greater social impact than did Jeff Astle's in the UK (despite similar coroner rulings), and why SRC debates are more pronounced in the US than elsewhere in the world.

In many ways children are at the 'sharp end' of this emergent *Brain Culture* because the child's brain is thought to have greater plasticity and thus early life experiences are thought to be particularly crucial in shaping futures. While changes in medicine, health, and *Brain Culture* shape sport's concussion crisis, social concern about youth and ageing is an additional and important mediating factor.

Childhood and ageing

Propelling sport's concussion crisis into public consciousness is its resonance with social concerns about the challenges of being at either end of the life-course. The regulatory changes (Chapter 3), the medical precaution (Chapter 4), and the focus of both behavioural science research and public health campaigns (Chapters 6 and 7) show how sustained is the focus on youth. But, equally, current concerns about SRC would be very differently expressed if it were not also for the connection with CTE and the potential exacerbation or early onset of age-related conditions such as dementia (Chapter 2). A perhaps unique feature of sport's concussion crisis, therefore, is the way in which these issues draw upon, become structured by, and ultimately feed back into cultural anxieties expressed about both the youngest and oldest in our society.

The significance of children in these debates extends far beyond the ethical jus-tification for paternalistic protection (see Chapter 5). This is indicated in the way that the future prosperity of children and sports are thought to be intertwined. On the one hand, as Messner and Musto (2014: 107) note, the idea that children represent the future of sport is 'front-and-center on the web sites of national sport organizations that fear the withering and eventual extinction of their sport if they fail to recruit and retain kids'. Children are literally and metaphorically depicted as society's future and the responsibility invested through this is matched by social expectations that result in the 'concerted cultivation' of youth (Messner and Musto 2014). 'Enrichment activities', of which physical exercise sits ahead of music and languages as the most popular form, require significant financial outlay and come to 'dominate family life and create enormous labour' (Vincent and Ball 2007: 1068). But parents make such sacrifices because they believe that sports participation will make their children more confident, improve their educational performance (Sabo and Veliz 2008), and so confer important advantages for later life. It is perhaps not surprising, therefore, that these attitudes inform the commitment to sport cultural norms (particularly among the young) which, in turn, fuels resistance to the restrictions on participation that uniquely flow from the diagnosis of concussion.

But the current relationship between youth and sport is part of a broader and temporally specific ideology of childhood. Meyer (2007) argues that a historical definition of children as small adults changed through a discourse of innocence and vulnerability developed in the Romanticism period (1800–1850).[2] Innocence leads childhood to be 'conceptualized as the cradle of the self' (Meyer 2007: 97), such that any harm experienced during this time is seen to be of paramount significance and potentially irreparable. The sense of vulnerability incorporates ideas about children being *physically* weak, *socially* limited in that they lack certain skills (and hence cannot give informed consent), and *structurally* disadvantaged in that they are less socially powerful than parents, teachers, etc. It is for this reason that a particularly compelling aspect of Ben Robinson's tragic death was the inability of his mother to intervene when she became concerned about his health (see Chapter 2).

Ideas about innocence and vulnerability combine to create an imperative for the adult protection of children. Children – and by implication children's brains – are seen to be at a heightened state of risk. In identifying the reasons behind the naming of the *Concussion Legacy Foundation*, the organization states that the word legacy 'was chosen to emphasize the fact that sports-related brain trauma in children leaves a permanent legacy in developing bodies . . . every hit to the head leaves a mark, or a legacy, on a child's future'.[3] It appears that the gravity of the problems facing the NFL following Omalu's 'discovery' of CTE were thrown into sharp relief by the realization that mothers might respond by withdrawing their children from football (Fainaru-Wada and Fainaru 2013). It has also been argued that the NFL have capitalized on such sentiment in backing youth concussion legislation in the US as a way of repairing the reputational damage inflicted by congressional hearings (Greenhow 2018).

Ironically, the 'innocence of childhood' ideology is in part responsible for the *creation* of sporting opportunities (e.g. the Pop Warner Football), which are now thought to expose children to unacceptable levels of risk (Laurendeau and Konecny 2015). Similarly, while the desire to nurture informs adult investments in the development of youth (sport), it also fuels the heightened concern over children's experiences of concussion. Children are positioned as too physically underdeveloped to withstand the forces that lead to concussion, as not having sufficient social skills to recognize the importance of withdrawing from sport when hurt, and thus in particular need of education and protection from the structural forces (coach coercion, compulsory physical education) that expose young people to the risk of concussion. Just as gender norms position the female child as *even more* innocent and vulnerable than her male counterpart, so sport's concussion crisis also entails greater concern about the vulnerability of girls relative to boys. Meyer's (2007: 99) contention that 'this rhetoric is so powerful that in fact *any* opinion can be justified by simply referring to children, and without having to explain *why* and *how* children justify it' reminds us of the claims made in both the concussion consensus statements and public health campaigns; there is no more compelling way to challenge existing practice than to be positioned as a protector of children. It is no coincidence, for instance, that all existing legal interventions (the Lystedt Laws, Rowan's Law) are named after children. But ironically these ideas ultimately lead us to neglect the voices of young people themselves and focus on altering rather than *understanding* their behaviour (see Chapter 7). Revelations about the potential dangers of taking part in sport feed back into these attitudes and fuel perceptions of the need to protect: if even our 'concerted cultivation' of youth exposes children to harm, can there be *any* context in which our children are not in need of our constant protection? In parallel with changing conceptions of health and the development of *Brain Culture*, the 'moral rhetoric of childhood' (Meyer 2007) underpins the central narratives of sport's concussion crisis.

Whereas these ideas explain why concerns are focussed towards the youngest end of the life-course spectrum, sport's concussion crisis also invokes concerns about the 'apocalyptic demography' said to stem from our ageing societies (Martin et al. 2009). Globally, it is estimated that dementia will cost approximately $1 trillion per year by 2030 and affect 80 million people by 2040 (Higgs and Gilleard 2017). Despite a general neglect of issues affecting the elderly, the sense that ageing is problematic – a burden caused by frail non-contributors with unsustainable health and social care costs – is widespread in media representations. Accounts which present frightening images of a brain-wasting disease as a kind of 'living death', and a panic-blame discourse which foregrounds the most extreme cases of dementia (in terms of both incapacity and early onset), demand urgent action to stem the 'tsunami', 'epidemic', or 'timebomb' (Peel 2014). Crucially, dementia is seen to limit not only the self-control of the individual, but also the capacity of carer-relatives to self-manage. As a consequence of its combined quantitative and qualitative parameters, dementia has become 'one of the global health priorities of our age . . . one of, if not the most feared aspects of growing old' (Hillman and Latimer 2017: 1).

The growing social concerns over dementia are a further manifestation of medicalization, as what was previously considered a 'normal' part of the ageing process has been repositioned as a medical problem (Davis 2004). But while pharmaceutical companies have been relatively successful in repositioning dementia as a medical condition rather than a normal part of ageing (as it has historically been viewed), the failure of the industry to produce a 'cure' has fuelled the trend towards identifying disease precursors and dementia prevention strategies (Higgs and Gilleard 2017). Although age overwhelmingly remains the primary risk factor, the main foci of dementia-related lifestyle medicine have been: poor diet; cardiovascular risk factors (such as tobacco and alcohol consumption, high blood pressure and cholesterol, etc.); cognitive stimulation (hence the aforementioned 'brain training' market); and the lack of physical exercise. Concern about concussion injuries locates sports participation – somewhat paradoxically given the perceived benefits of exercise – on this broader agenda.

The prominence of these social processes provides part of the explanation for the bias towards issues relating to CTE and the general sense of fear propagated in the media (see Chapter 3). The focus on athletes – e.g. Webster, Astle, Boogard, Duerson – provides some of the *most* atypical and *severe* cases and thus sits comfortably with the broader cultural representation of dementia. The panic–blame discourse appears in relation to the duty (and/or denial) of sport governing bodies to address the potential harms of head injuries. Campaigns, for example, to ban heading in soccer, replicate the pattern of risk profiling and 'faddy avoidance' tactics (Peel, 2014) evident in the wider response to ageing and dementia. In this sense, rather than sport being a potential cause of dementia, social concerns about dementia could be said to be a *cause* of sport's concussion crisis.

Before we move to consider how the major social processes shaping contemporary sport influence this cultural crisis, we must finally consider the relationship between ageing and gender. Dementia affects more women than men by a ratio of almost 2:1 (Alzheimer's Society 2014). But sport's particularly gendered history raises serious questions about whether participation could be a significant 'cause' of longer-term neurocognitive decline across the population (overall, what proportion of those currently diagnosed with dementia would have played tackle football or have regularly headed a ball?). The media's focus on extreme cases skews our appreciation of this, for while we have seen that heightened concerns are expressed in relation to the risk of concussion for girls, the vast majority of high-profile cases relate directly to males (Pat Summit, a US college basketball coach being a notable exception). Contemporary concerns about dementia are effectively fuelled by the inclusion of these cases as they focus on younger, male 'victims' and reach out to younger, male audiences in a way that ageing-related stories rarely do. Sport's concussion crisis is not just the outcome of cultural anxieties about ageing and dementia, it provides cases which serve to amplify these broader social processes.

Sport

While changes to medicine/health and perceptions of childhood/ageing fundamentally structure sport's concussion crisis, the way modern sport is organized and experienced is the proverbial 'elephant in the room'. There are, perhaps, four particularly important factors: the pacification of sport; commercialization; nationalism and globalization; and the advancement of what was earlier described as the sport–health ideology.

Broadly speaking, modern sport developed in Britain around the mid-1700s. This process was first evident in sports such as boxing, cricket, golf, and horse-racing and entailed relatively loosely defined and structured 'folk games' becoming organized through rules which were written down and enforced by a third party (referee, umpire, etc.). The process was linked to broader social structural changes which do not need to be discussed here (see e.g., Malcolm and Haut 2018), but importantly it involved many of the more violent aspects of folk games being phased out. A wider range of such rule-bound, standardized, and relatively pacified sports developed through the 1800s (notably association and rugby football) and were diffused around the globe (hence American and Australian Rules football) via the extensive networks of the formal and informal British Empire. It was in this context that equality (of opportunity) became a more explicit guiding principle.

In trying to understand why these types of activities became socially valued, Elias and Dunning (1986) propose the 'quest for excitement' thesis. They argue that as societies become more regulated, the popularity of sports rests on their capacity to provide a sphere of social life in which participants experience a 'controlled de-controlling of emotional controls'. Messner (1992) provides a compatible argument: the development of modern sport in the US was a response to the end of the American frontier and the greater routinization of life for those in urban industrial environments. Notably, however, Messner gives particular emphasis to the role of masculinity. Modern sports, he argues, were developed in response to the perceived feminization of childhood and as a means through which to foster traditional masculine behaviours which had developed more 'naturally' in the relatively 'uncontrolled' frontier societies.

Both these ideas help explain why many sports (and particularly those that feature prominently in sport's concussion crisis) involve physical contact that would be deemed illegal in other social settings, and why we experience and express emotions in heightened and more intense ways than we do in 'everyday' life. Part of the continuing appeal of sports is that they provide an antidote to the emotional routine of contemporary living. While perhaps beyond the remit of the CISG consensus statements, there is a logic to the stated concerns about *preserving* the competitive/aggressive 'essence' of sport (see Chapter 4).

Consequently, and contrary to many popular portrayals of sport and American and rugby football in particular, these activities are now much less violent than their predecessors were. However, our likelihood of experiencing injury while taking part remains *relatively* high when compared to other pastimes. In parallel, the continued commitment to equality has democratized participation across gender, class, etc., thereby exposing a wider population to these relative dangers.

Sport's concussion crisis relates to both of these points. First, the spill-over effect fundamental to a cultural crisis is in part driven by the idea that these activities could and should be open to all, not just the more 'resilient' social classes and gender. Sport's first concussion crisis (Harrison 2014), it should be remembered, related primarily to US (male) college football. Second, concerns about SRC are in many ways the result of the reduction in other types of injuries incurred during sport rather than a consequence of the increasing dangers of these sports per se. For instance, Freitag et al. (2015) cite a 97 per cent reduction in scrum injuries in rugby union in New Zealand, and Quarrie et al. (2017: 1138) argue that 'permanently disabling rugby injuries to children are very rare events'. The displacement of injury can be seen in boxing, where the introduction of gloves has been effective in reducing cuts to the head and hands but has had the unintended but potential consequence of increasing incidence of brain injury (Sheard 2003). Concussion has, in many ways, either become the primary concern as other dangers have been addressed or become more prevalent due to attempts to eliminate other types of injury. At the same time, the quest for excitement explains why participants in the sports community are continually resistant to the regulation of concussion which forces their withdrawal from activities. Sports participation is rarely (only) about health, and motives for participation are often much more about generating excitement and identity formation.

A second sport-related development informing our understanding of sport's concussion crisis is commercialization. Again this is manifest in a number of ways. First, and largely due to the capacity of sport to engage the emotions as described previously, vast sums of money now rest on the management of sports events. With media and sponsorship income eclipsing the value of gate receipts, not only do we see the owners and controllers having deeply vested interests in sport's continued smooth functioning, but we see a redefinition of the relationship between these organizations and sports fans/consumers. The corruption scandals involving global bodies such as FIFA and the International Olympic Committee (IOC), and the ownership of sports teams by economic elites, lead to increasing levels of scepticism about the propriety and motives of sports administrators and the degree to which athletes might be exploited for economic gain. As these relationships become more conflictual/antagonistic, so the cultural industry's definition of 'newsworthiness' changes; for example, the practices of sports organizations like the NFL that have been depicted as denial (Fainaru-Wada and Fainaru 2013). Similar, but considerably less substantiated claims, have been made in relation to the AFL (Carlisle 2018), the Football Association (FA), and the Professional Footballers' Association in England.[4]

Second, the quest for commercially rewarded (and/or nationally prestigious victory), has fuelled the rational pursuit of enhanced athletic performance. As a consequence, sport has become, 'an intensive, exhaustive occupation where athletes are fully embroiled in sophisticated training regimes utilizing scientifically developed technologies that create long-term physiological and personality changes as they progress through the high-stakes, "winner-takes-all" road to the pinnacle of world-class sport' (Beamish and Ritchie 2006: 8). This is most evident in the NFL and elite rugby union/league where physical power is vital to the outcome of contests, but it is equally true across the other sports discussed here. Indicatively, whilst 20 years ago research on SRC was thought to be limited due to the lack of comparability with car-related head injury, the impacts experienced in sport today are routinely compared to road traffic accidents. The combination of scientific methods and the desire for continuous improvement leads sports organizations and cultures to develop performers who extend our understanding of the limits of human capabilities.

At the intersection of commercialization and the development of these super-human beings is celebrity culture (Marshall 1997). Contemporary fascinations with celebrity have been attributed to a desire to foster emotional closeness in response to the decline of traditional forms of social bonding (e.g. religion) and increasingly individualized societies (Rojek 2001). Consequently, these 'extraordinary' individuals are propelled into the public realm, and the growth in media coverage enables 'fans' to have far greater access to information about elite sports performers than ever before. The private and public spheres become increasingly blurred, and routinely we receive/expect to hear the minutia of athletes' lives. While physically, economically, and experientially these sports stars are far further divorced from the 'ordinary' person than they ever have been, the perception is often rather different.

Thus, although CTE emerged as an occupationally specific condition, the *Intimate Strangers* (Schickel 1997) created by celebrity culture makes 'ordinary' people feel that the dangers of elite sports participation apply in a relatively direct way to themselves. While Quarrie et al. (2017) argue that the absence of reliable data about the incidence, impact, and experience of concussion leads people to extrapolate what they see via the media and assume it to be relevant across the population, this is part of a wider yet flawed perception. Commercialization and celebrity culture create both a separation and perceived closeness that spreads concerns about SRC. Where once retired sports star could easily fade from public view, the powerful elements of nostalgia in the culture of sports celebrity provide ex-performers with a series of 're-births' (Whannel 2002). Our interest in, and exposure to, the longer-term mental health of retired athletes is a logical and inevitable extension of celebrity culture. The concerns about the incidence of dementia among England's World Cup winning team is a striking example.

A third key social process is the politicization of sports which have become an increasingly significant forum for international status competition. In combination with the pacification of social life, modern sport has always reflected George Orwell's maxim of 'war minus the shooting'. However, the globalization of media coverage means that the potential value of using sports events for national ends is greater than ever before. This is most clearly expressed in terms of the competition to host sport mega-events such as the Olympic Games. But a rising and related trend has also been the militarization of major domestic sports events. As Butterworth (2017: 2) argues, 'military references are routine components in broadcasts and live events' such that the 'entanglements' of sport and the military are 'too numerous to mention'. Critical questioning of the military is deemed unpatriotic (Kelly 2012) and hence, as noted in Chapter 3, a military connection has been specifically mobilized in the NFL's public relations to construct an anti-politics message which serves to overshadow concerns about concussion and CTE as a labour issue (Brayton et al. 2019; Benson 2017). The frequent comparison between post-concussive syndrome and PTSD further extends this narrative and serves to capitalize on the post-9/11 valorization of those who represent the nation in both real and proxy wars. Thus, sport has become an increasingly useful tool for states to generate more coherent expressions of national identity within our ever more globalized world.

The juxtaposition of globalization and nationalism explains why sport's concussion crisis is both the first sports injury crisis to have global reach, yet manifests in nationally specific ways. Briefly stated, SRC concerns have been most pronounced in the national sports of the respective nations. While conscious that the identification of a particular national sport is more complicated than this suggests (see, e.g. Bairner 2001), it is far from coincidental that it is American football, ice hockey, the AFL, and rugby union that are the main foci of sport's concussion crisis in the US, Canada, Australia, and New Zealand, respectively.[5] Of course, each of these sports is relatively violent (which, in turn, relates back to our continued 'quest for excitement' and notions of masculinity), but the prominence of SRC concerns in soccer in both Britain and to a lesser extent Italy shows how national self-image mediates concussion debates beyond any simple direct correlation with a particular sport's injury rates. It also explains why resistance to the more conservative voices in sports concussion crisis are so strong; the debates largely occur within and mobilize the defence of national self-image. Indicatively, the fact that the most significant soccer rule changes have occurred in the US relates not simply to the heightened level of public concern over concussion in North America, but also to soccer's relatively marginal status in that context. The importance of national identity in the contemporary world (and modern sport) also provides an explanation why, despite decades of relatively reliable empirical evidence of harm, public outcry about concussion in boxing and other combat sports remains relatively muted. These 'fighters' are rarely and much less directly associated with sporting nationalism.

The fourth sport-related development that contributes to the concussion crisis is the growing cultural and political commitment to the sport-health ideology. While these ideas have a long history, recent developments have strengthened their resonance. Physical activity is now one of the 'big four' themes of health promotion (alongside alcohol, food consumption, and tobacco), with exercise even claimed to be 'today's best buy in public health' (AMRC 2015). Indicative of the contemporary commitment to the sport-health ideology is the development of the Exercise is Medicine programme, now adopted in 39 nations across the globe (Lobelo et al. 2014). Frequently sport is seen as the best or *only* way that the so-called Obesity Epidemic (Gard and Wright 2004) can be reversed.

There are a number of problems with drawing such a direct correlation between exercise and health, and there are a number of broader societal considerations which help us to understand why the sport-health ideology remains both so pervasive and resilient (Malcolm 2017; Malcolm and Pullen 2018). The central point here, however, is that political elites (and public opinion) are fundamentally wedded to the idea that more physical activity (which, in reality is often conflated with sports participation) is a vital strategy for improving population health and reducing state medical costs. As previously noted, exercising for health has become positioned as a socially responsible act. Once again, the rhetoric of childhood creates a disproportionate focus is place on the behaviours and futures of children (McDermott 2007). Equally those responsible for the organization and administration of sport are receptive to these ideas because, especially in times of declining state subsidy, the sport-health ideology provides a compelling rationale for continued funding. In the current climate, sport becomes projected as having 'unquestioned benefits' for health (Calderwood et al. 2016), while raising issues about the potential of sport to create ill-health challenges a wide range of vested interests (see Chapter 7).

The strengthening of the sport-health ideology links with the changing social conceptualization of health noted previously. In this context, exercising is seen as a virtuous behaviour, a proactive and responsible form of citizenship. But an inevitable consequence of the social status accrued from such activities is that it becomes mobilized in the defence individuals may mount in relation to their autonomy to participate in sport. The logic expressed is that if I am doing something so socially responsible, why would my decisions about exercising be subject to external regulation (see Chapter 6)? While, the potential issues related to CTE makes such logic problematic, ultimately sport's concussion crisis must be understood in relation to the complexities of the sport-health ideology being challenged by evidence of the health-harming consequences of sport.

Conclusion

The purpose of this chapter has been to explore what sport's concussion crisis tells us about the societies in which we live. The review has identified a number of social processes which converge in relation to brain injury. As we have seen, we live in societies which: are both relatively medicalized yet contain considerable scepticism about the efficacy of modern medicine; have come to evaluate 'health' in relation to one's relative independence from health professionals; and see 'fitness' as a fundamental indicator of our capacity for bodily self-control and hence responsible citizenship. This in turn has led to the positioning of lifestyle and the brain-maintenance as the fundamental components of good health, a combination which draws our attention to the perceived importance of childhood in setting the template for life-long health, and the ultimate expression of this being seen in our neurocognitive capacity when older. To be recognized as responsible citizens it is our duty to consider what we do – and how we structure children's lives – to optimize the longer-term impact on a condition we particularly fear: dementia. At the heart of sport's concussion crisis is the paradox that the health imperative compels us to exercise which, we now fear, could ultimately destroy our health in the way we most fear and which we see as defining our essence as humans.

While these processes significantly impact on how we come to view sport (and exercise) as a tool for health self-management in its current holistic sense (physical, mental, and social development), these perceptions are almost entirely at odds with the processes of commericialization, corporatization, globalization, nationalism, militarism, etc., that appear dominant in structuring elite sport. Sport is, at one and the same time, developing an elite level model that is increasingly distant from the public's lived experience and becoming positioned as fundamental to our own well-being such that our participation is expected across the life course. These elements provide the underlying contradictions that create the cultural divide evident in sport's concussion crisis. They combine to create the forces which, so far, have made resolution beyond reach.

Notes

1 www.prnewswire.com/news-releases/global-cognitive-assessment-and-training-market
    -2017-2021-aging-population-increasing-awareness-for-brain-fitness–advancement-i
    n-technology-drive-the-806-billion-market—research-and-markets-300443424.html
2 Perhaps not uncoincidentally, Mill's ideas about the paternalistic exemptions to the
    sovereignty of individual liberty (idiots or infants), were first published in 1859.

3 https://concussionfoundation.org/
4 www.independent.co.uk/sport/football/premier-league/pfa-chief-executive-gordon-ta
   ylor-resign-full-open-review-salary-a8644876.html Accessed 18 February 2019.
5 The exception here is Ireland, where SRC is a greater concern in rugby union than
   Gaelic games. It should be noted, however, that rugby union largely unites the island of
   Ireland, in a way that Gaelic games separates the South from (most of) the North.

References

Alzheimer's Society (2014). *Dementia UK: Update*. London: Alzheimer's Society.
AMRC (2015) *Exercise: The Miracle Cure and the Role of the Doctor in Promoting it*. London: Academy of Medical Royal Colleges.
Aronowitz, R. (2009) 'The converged experience of risk and disease', *The Milbank Quarterly*, 87(2): 417–442.
Bachynski, K. (2019) '"The duty of their elders": doctors, coaches, and the framing of youth football's health risks, 1950s–1960s', *Journal of the History of Medicine and Allied Sciences*, 74 (2): 167–191.
Bairner, A. (2001) *Sport, Nationalism, and Globalization*. New York: SUNY Press.
Bauman, Z. (2000) *Liquid Modernity*. Cambridge: Polity Press.
Beamish, R. and Ritchie, I. (2006) *Fastest, Highest, Strongest: A Critique of High Performance Sport*. London: Routledge.
Benson, P. (2017) 'Big football: corporate social responsibility and the culture and color of injury in America's most popular sport', *Journal of Sport & Social Issues*, 41(4): 307–334.
Brayton, S., Helstien, M., Ramsey, M., and Rickards, N. (2019) 'Exploring the missing link between the concussion "crisis" and labor politics in professional sports', *Communication and Sport*, 7(1): 110–131.
Butterworth, M. (2017) 'Sport and militarism: An introduction to a global phenomenon', in M. Butterworth (ed.), *Sport and Militarism: Contemporary Global Perspectives*, London: Routledge, 1–13.
Calderwood, C., Murray, A., and Stewart, W. (2016) 'Turning people into couch potatoes is not the cure for sports concussion', *British Journal of Sports Medicine*, 50(4): 200–201.
Cant, S. and Sharma, U. (1999) *A New Medical Pluralism? Alternative Medicine, Doctors, Patients and the State*. London: UCL Press.
Carlisle, W. (2018) 'The AFL's concussion problem: is the league running interference on the damage concussion can cause?' www.themonthly.com.au/issue/2018/september/1535724000/wendy-carlisle/afl-s-concussion-problem
Conrad, P. (1992) 'Medicalization and social control', *Annual Review of Sociology*, 18: 209–232.
Crawford, R. (1980) 'Healthism and the medicalization of everyday life', *International Journal of Health Services*, 10(3): 365–388.
Davis, D. (2004). Dementia: sociological and philosophical constructions. *Social Science & Medicine*, 58: 369–378.
Elias, N. (2000) *The Civilizing Process: Sociogenetic and Psychogenetic Investigations*. Oxford: Blackwell (3rd edition).
Elias, N. and Dunning, E. (1986) *Quest for Excitement: Sport and Leisure in the Civilising Process*. Blackwell: Oxford.
Fainaru-Wada, M., and Fainaru, S. (2013) *League of Denial*. New York: Crown Business.
Fox, R.C. (2000) 'Medical uncertainty revisited', in G.L. Albrecht, R. Fitzpatrick and S.C. Scrimshaw (eds.), *The Handbook of Social Studies in Health and Medicine*, London: SAGE, 409–425.

Freitag, A., Kirkwood, G., Pollock, A.M. (2015a) 'Rugby injury surveillance and prevention programmes: are they effective?', *British Medical Journal*, 350: h1587.

Gale, N. (2011) 'From body-talk to body-stories: body work in complementary and alternative medicine', *Sociology of Health and Illness*, 33(2): 237–251.

Gard, M. and Wright, J. (2004) *The Obesity Epidemic: Science, Morality and Ideology*. London: Routledge.

Glassner, B. (1990) 'Fit for postmodern selfhood', in H. Becker and M. McCall (eds.) *Symbolic Interactionism and Cultural Studies*, Chicago, IL: Chicago University Press.

Greenhow, A. (2018) *Why the Brain Matters: Regulating Concussion in Australian Sport*. Unpublished PhD thesis, Monash University, Melbourne Australia.

Harrison, E. (2014) 'The first concussion crisis: head injury and evidence in early American football', *American Journal of Public Health*, 104(5): 822–833.

Higgs, P. and Gilleard, C. (2017). 'Ageing, dementia and the social mind: past, present and future perspectives', *Sociology of Health & Illness*, 39(2): 175–181.

Hillman, A. and Latimer, J. (2017). 'Cultural representations of dementia', *Plos Medicine*, 14 (3):e102274.

Huber, M., Knotternus, J.A., Green., L. et al. (2011) 'How should we define health?' *British Medical Journal*, 343: d4163. doi:10.1136/bmj.d4163.

Johnson Thornton, D. (2011) *Brain Culture: Neuroscience and Popular Media*. New Brunswick, NJ: Rutgers University Press.

Kelly, J. (2012) 'Popular culture, sport and the 'hero'-fication of British militarism', *Sociology*, 47(4): 722–738.

Laurendeau, J. and Konecny, D. (2015) 'Where is childhood? In conversation with Messner and Musto', *Sociology of Sport Journal*, 32: 332–344.

Lobelo, F., Stoutenberg, M. and Hutber, A. (2014) 'The Exercise Is Medicine global health initiative: a 2014 update', *British Journal of Sports Medicine*, 48(22): 1627–1633.

Lupton, D. (1995) *The Imperative of Health. Public Health and the Regulated Body*. London: SAGE.

Malcolm, D. (2017) *Sport, Medicine and Health: The Medicalization of Sport?* London: Routledge.

Malcolm, D. (2019) 'Concussion, chronic traumatic encephalopathy, and the medicalization of sport', in M. Ventresca and M. Macdonald (eds.), *Brain Injury in Sport*, New York: Routledge.

Malcolm, D. and Haut, J. (2018) 'The development of modern sport: sportization and civilizing processes', in D. Malcolm and P. Velija (eds.) *Figurational Research in Sport, Leisure and Health*, London: Routledge, 23–33.

Malcolm, D. and Pullen, E. (2018) 'Is exercise medicine?', in L. Mansfield, J. Piggin, and M. Weed (eds.), *Handbook of Physical Activity: Policy, Politics and Practice*, London: Routledge, 49–60.

Marshall, P.D. (1997) *Celebrity and Power: Fame in Contemporary Culture*. Minneapolis: University of Minnesota Press.

Martin, R., Williams, C., and O'Neill, D. (2009). 'Retrospective analysis of attitudes to ageing in the Economist: apocalyptic demography for opinion formers', *British Medical Journal*, 339: b4914.

McDermott, L. (2007) 'A governmental analysis of children "at risk" in a world of physical inactivity and obesity epidemics', *Sociology of Sport Journal*, 24: 302–324.

Messner, M. (1992) *Power at Play: Sport and the Problems of Masculinity*, Boston, MA: Beacon Press.

Messner, M. and Musto, M. (2014) 'Where are the kids?', *Sociology of Sport Journal*, 31: 102–122.

Meyer, A. (2007) 'The moral rhetoric of childhood', *Childhood*, 14(1): 85–104.

Peel, E. (2014). "'The living death of Alzheimer's" versus "Take a walk to keep dementia at bay": representations of dementia in the print media and carer discourse', *Sociology of Health & Illness*, 36(6): 885–901.

Quarrie, K., Brookes, J., Burger, N., Hume, P., and Jackson, S. (2017) 'Facts and values: on the acceptability of risks in children's sport using the example of rugby: a narrative review', *British Journal of Sports Medicine*, 51: 1134–1139.

Rojek, C. (2001) *Celebrity*. London: Reaktion Books.

Sabo, D. and Veliz, P. (2008) *Youth Sport in America*. New York: Women's Sports Foundation.

Schickel, R. (1997) *Intimate Strangers: The Culture of Celebrity in America*. Chicago, IL: Ivan R. Dee.

Sheard, K. (2003) 'Boxing in the western civilizing process', in E. Dunning, D. Malcolm, and I. Waddington (eds.), *Sport Histories: Figurational Studies of the Development of Modern Sports*, London: Routledge, 15–30.

Vincent, C. and Ball, S. (2007) '"Making up" the middle-class child: families, activities and class dispositions', *Sociology*, 41(6): 1061–1077.

Whannel, G. (2002) *Media Sport Stars: Masculinities and Moralities*. London: Routledge.

9

THE FUTURE

It was going mad on Twitter. Ash read the calls for new rules and harsher punishments, and accusations that 'they' weren't taking concussion seriously. But the more people argued, the further apart the sides seemed to get. 'Surely there's a solution to all this?'

While the comparison with 'big tobacco' has featured prominently in sport's concussion crisis, a perhaps better analogy would be contemporary debates about climate change. Those labelled 'deniers' effectively take a 'very "high proof" position on consensus and expertise' (Sismondo 2017: 5), arguing that there is insufficient evidence that human behaviour is causing global temperatures to rise. This is akin to one half of the concussion debate which queries the degree of harm sports participants are exposed to and the strength of the causal link to CTE. On the other side of the climate change debate lies the scientifically orthodox position that action is urgently required to save humanity from disaster, much as do those who position SRC as an epidemic in their attempts to invoke more precautionary behaviours and greater regulatory change. Climate change debates are also characterized by claims of conspiracy in the representation of scientific data. Here, the claims made about 'erroneous and misleading' portrayals of the risks of SRI mirror the 2009 'Climategate' scandal (Fuller 2018) in which leading UK researchers were exposed as colluding to create the appearance of scientific consensus.

The climate change comparison is also useful in that it directs us to what has come to be called the post-truth condition. Post-truth is a recently developed term, first defined in the 2016 Oxford English Dictionary as 'relating to or denoting circumstances in which objective facts are less influential in shaping public opinion than appeals to emotion and personal belief'. While the mix of politics and science is 'endemic to the history of Western thought' (Fuller 2018: 181), unique to the contemporary landscape is the degree of democratization of knowledge fostered by the expansion and diversification of media outlets, and the development of 'social media echo chambers' (Lockie 2017: 2). The essential continuity in the post-truth condition is that the established scientific community positions a new and anti-establishment group as irrationally challenging the 'facts', and the newcomers respond by 'going meta', in other words, attempting to switch the rules of the debate to more favourable terrain (Fuller 2018: 3).

The characteristics of the post-truth condition are also writ large in sport's concussion crisis. While the battle lines between science and the respective sides in sport's concussion crisis are less clear, debates over whether epidemiological data over- or underestimate the true incidence of concussion, and whether media reporting either sensationalizes concussion or obscures some fundamental issues related to organizational malpractice, illustrate how the post-truth condition is characterized by 'the view that reality is fundamentally different from what most people think' (Fuller 2018: 1). The idea that there are such things as 'undiagnosed' concussions, that individuals with no medical training can make a self-diagnosis, or that athletes might make that diagnosis simply by looking at their teammates (see Chapter 6) is indicative of the kind of confusion on which post-truth thrives. The Hollywood dramatization of the work of Bennet Omalu represents a more radical, individual, and 'asocial' intervention than a historical perspective recognizing the pre-existing lay and scientific knowledge can sustain, but equally one sees how the work of the scientific establishment (through the Concussion in Sport Group consensus statements) shows evidence of the 'feats of fudging, complicating, back-tracking and all round "adhockery" that the orthodoxy must routinely perform to show that it is getting closer to the truth' (Fuller 2018: 5). When a group of pre-eminent UK neuroscientists published a letter in the *Lancet* calling for 'balance' in the reporting of CTE (Stewart et al. 2019), its lead author (the UK's equivalent of Ann McKee) took to *Twitter* to highlight what were essentially allegations of 'fake news' from critics who felt that the case for the existence and causation of CTE had been queried.

In sport's concussion crisis, neither side has an *a priori* claim to be representing the 'truth' or is immune from invoking emotion to persuade others. Indeed, a unique aspect of the concussion crisis (unique to sport that is) is that as a consequence of the NFL's previous questioning of both the prevalence and significance of head injury, and continued debates about the 'proof' of a causal link between SRC and longer-term neurological decline, the act of simply saying that there is uncertainty over concussion has itself become politically contentious. While earlier Paul McCrory was 'accredited' with playing a significant role in formalizing and standardizing biomedical knowledge about SRC, more recently his continued prominence in the CISG consensus statements has led to claims that he is a major proponent of CTE-scepticism, too closely aligned with the vested interests of sports organizations, and, subsequently, an obstacle to more radical change (Carlisle 2018). Indicative of the fluidity of positions within the post-truth condition was President Trump's volte face about concussion around the 2019 Super Bowl, when he reversed his previous stance of 'sport going soft' by expressing his discomfort at the thought of his son playing American football.

These comments illustrate how sport's concussion crisis, like our post-truth condition more generally, is characterized by deep schisms and rapidly changing 'rules of the game'. How, then, can the deeply ingrained divisions of this cultural crisis be resolved? We focus on three particular areas of development: biomedical or technically based solutions; game-related solutions; and cultural change. Given that, from the outset, I have argued that sport's concussion crisis must be considered a cultural, rather than simply a biomedical or sporting phenomenon, it logically follows that I see the greatest potential for resolution laying in the cultural domain.

Biotechnical solutions

Biotechnical solutions to sport's concussion crisis focus on the enhancement of diagnostic tools, treatment, and preventative equipment. As noted in Chapter 4, we start from a low base of accepted scientific knowledge but, rather than creating opportunities, this merely serves to compound the significant barriers each will continue to face.

For instance, while sports have variously experimented with 'concussion spotters', independent doctors, and the use of technology such as 'hawkeye' (a movement tracking system) to detect concussions (Greenhow 2018), the development of a diagnostic biomarker (i.e. blood, saliva, or urine) is particularly keenly awaited. Yet as no diagnostic test is 100 per cent accurate, debates about the acceptable levels of sensitivity and specificity (the number of false positives or negatives) will be ongoing. Moreover, will the presence of signs traditionally associated with concussion (e.g. loss of consciousness) be disregarded if a diagnostic test is negative? Would a more 'accurate' diagnostic tool eliminate second impact syndrome (SIS), the mechanisms of which we currently do not understand? Indeed, the notion of a single diagnostic tool implies that existing theories about gender and age as 'modifying factors' for concussion may be rejected, yet it is unlikely that science alone will shift these deeply socially rooted concerns. The areas of uncertainty in concussion science are so broad that no single innovation will remove the suspicions which perpetuate the broader crisis.

Second, while future biotechnical interventions may improve the capacity of medicine to treat those with concussion, symptoms are so diffuse and develop over such varying timespans that it is difficult to know the extent of what would constitute 'cure'. One of the unique features of SRC is that the presence of symptoms is so divorced from the conditions that cause concern. Is it enough to resolve immediately displayed symptoms, or post-concussive syndrome, or longer-term neurological decline?

Related to this would be the development of a clearer understanding of the link between sport and longer-term developing neurological conditions such as CTE and ALS. Evidence of no or minimal links would, of course, de-escalate sport's concussion crisis, whereas compelling and incontrovertible evidence might raise existential questions for certain sports forms. But the most likely scenario is the most problematic scenario; that evidence will develop that continues to show the link as ambiguous. In this regard important considerations will be: which aspects of sport, or particular sporting practices, increase the risk of developing longer-term conditions? Is the development of these conditions consigned to just a few or all sports? What non-sport activities contribute to the development of these conditions? The questions that will ultimately need to be answered are, however, social: what, and how many, aspects of social life can we eliminate and yet retain an existence which people find tolerable if not pleasurable? Consequently, the development of this scientific knowledge will lead to the positing of questions potentially just as problematic as sport's current concussion crisis.

Third, while protective equipment innovations have focussed on improving helmet design, there is no known exact correlation between impact forces and concussion, with no absolute force threshold below which SRCs are eliminated or above which SRC inevitably occurs. We do not know what particular forces lead to which symptomatic outcomes (e.g. amnesia, disorientation, loss of consciousness). Moreover, while helmets have been effectively developed to absorb impact forces, because energy is displaced rather than neutralized there is always a danger that the risk of injury is similarly referred. This, for instance, is a concern over the use of headguards in boxing. Although they effectively reduce cuts, do they make the head heavier and so increase the risk of injury to the relatively free-floating brain within the skull?

Regardless of intervention type, implementation always represents an overarching challenge for biotechnical solutions. Indeed, if currently the base of concussion science is low, the effective implementation of existing regulations should perhaps be an even greater concern. Moreover, interventions will need to be available across the spectrum of sporting performance rather than the preserve of elite athletes. Spectators already see clinicians returning players to games after exhibiting some of the symptoms commonly associated with concussion, and this frequently becomes the focus of media debates about concussion guidelines. Interventions that are only available to the minority will perpetuate divisions and debates.

Implementation would further require an assessment of risk compensation behaviours, because people who feel 'safer' frequently take more risks. But the nature of modern sport dictates that every facet of the game (including new protective equipment) becomes an opportunity for competitive advantage. For instance, the introduction of protective equipment when rugby union became professional was perceived to have increased injury rates (Malcolm et al. 2004), while in the NFL particularly effective helmets have made for particularly effective weapons, contributing to particularly high rates of injury.

Finally, technological solutions must sit within the existing issues relating to patient management. In reality we already have diagnostic criteria which recognize a holistic set of signs and symptoms, do not require esoteric medical skills, and are relatively widely available and quick to apply (if one employs the precautionary stance of withdrawing all those *suspected* of being concussed). Resistance to existing diagnostic tools comes from concerns about balancing the potential impact on sport performance. Ultimately, however, where to draw the precautionary line is a cultural rather than biotechnical question.

Compounding all these issues is the evidence that the development of biotechnical interventions tends to lead to a reconceptualization of the condition they are designed to identify/treat (Timmermans and Buchbinder 2012). Introducing new diagnoses or treatments effectively constitutes a new form of 'experiment' which, when deployed in more varied contexts, *will* reveal new findings and create new understandings of this and related conditions. This is the normal process of scientific refinement and development (for instance, screening for diabetes has led to the identification of pre-diabetic cases). Moreover, this has already happened through revisions to the understanding of SRC in the last 20 years, a process I termed *concussion inflation* (see Chapter 4). De-medicalization processes are possible, but the diagnosis, treatment, and prevention of concussion is likely to be incremental rather than definitive, and likely to be contested along the way by the different concussion communities.

Game-related solutions

A second set of solutions focus on the tighter regulation of sport. First, there are suggestions for rule changes to be implemented to constrain age-group practices. In addition to the US prohibition of heading in youth soccer and campaigns for the banning of tackling in rugby in schools, Cantu and Hyman (2012) have argued for age-group restrictions on tackle football and body-checking in ice hockey and on various forms of striking (to the body or head) in MMA. Second, there are suggestions for rule changes across individual sports. For instance, Caron and Bloom (2015) propose five rule changes to improve player health and safety in ice hockey (e.g. increasing the width of the ice and the length of suspensions, the elimination of fighting, the greater accountability of owners). Similarly, Cantu and Hyman (2012) argue that helmets should be made mandatory in field hockey and girls' lacrosse (to standardize with the men's game), that baseball helmets should have chin straps, and that use of the head-first slide to base should be restricted. Third, there are calls for the abolition of sports in their entirety. Currently few combat sports are prohibited (e.g. bare-knuckle fighting, though not necessarily due to concussion concerns), but medical associations and brain injury campaign groups continue to petition for the prohibition of (other) combat sports and so pose this existential threat to certain activities.

While it is important to recognize that any blanket refusal to consider rule changes is problematic from both a historical and logical standpoint, the boundaries of possible change are not limitless. Sports have continually changed rules, sometimes evoked to retain a tension balance between attack and defence (and so generate excitement), and sometimes to moderate violence and injury. At times these processes are rapid and easily identified, while at other times they are more organic and incremental. Sport's concussion crisis fosters an environment in which more radical and injury-related changes are likely but claims that any individual rule change would undermine the 'essence' of a sport – in other words, pose an axiological threat – are alarmist. If the social significance of sport in modern societies relates to a quest for excitement, then people will likely continue to seek out (and find) those activities which engender a relative de-routinization of the 'norms' of social and emotional controls. The development of MMA is indicative of this process. Socially determined and historically variable upper and lower thresholds of violence and 'staleness' facilitate a quest for excitement and so shape the socially acceptable parameters of sports (Sanchez Garcia and Malcolm 2010).

That said, the problems with each of the three specific types of rule change are such that they cannot provide a total solution. Specifically, prohibition is always problematic from a libertarian ethical viewpoint. Even with a relatively high degree of medical consensus, and rationales for the distinctive character of combat sports, abolition campaigns have been resisted. Moreover, even if the prohibition of fighting sports was achieved, this *alone* would not end debates over SRCs which, as noted, embrace an ever-expanding set of sporting activities. And yet, conversely, a more comprehensive ban of sports is also unlikely as the differences between other conflict and contact sports are much less clear, and on these issues the medical community is even less united. Either way, it would be difficult to maintain the case for prohibition, when such 'self-harming' activities as smoking tobacco are legal.

Second, the fundamental problem with age-group regulation is that the cut-off point is always contestable. While there appears to be a broad-brush acceptance of the principles of paternalism (all sides of the concussion debate argue for the more conservative treatment of children), this largely shows the predominance of emotion over evidence. Moreover, definitions of child/adulthood are culturally determined and geographically varied, creating further difficulties when implementing an essentially 'task oriented' approach to competence. Working out who is capable of assessing what kind of risks will be a contentious process. Finally, a problem that stems from implementing such discrete rule changes is that, so far, they have largely been seen by critics as tokenistic. Minor changes are unlikely to generate the degree of change required to resolve cultural crisis.

An additional set of 'game-related' proposals target sport's regulators. These suggestions include calls for a stronger emphasis on implementation and ensuring the accountability of those responsible for enforcing concussion harm reduction policies (e.g. Cantu and Hyman, 2012; Partridge 2014). Yet such is the lack of confidence in sports governing bodies to put their 'houses in order' that others propose that even concussion awareness programmes should be passed to a neutral or non-sport agency (Goldberg 2013). This would have the merit of complying with calls for a more coordinated approach across sports, the logic being that participants (and clinicians) rarely sit in the kind of isolation that the distinct boundaries between sports governing bodies create, and that different regulations cause confusion, scepticism, and fuel non-compliance. Yet a more coordinated approach may be resisted by those who argue that it is unreasonable to treat equally the very different types of activity embroiled in the concussion crisis (e.g. from boxing to baseball). Greater state or external regulation is likely to be resisted by those wishing to preserve the traditional relative autonomy of sports governance.

A final proposal is to rethink the paradigmatic assumptions of existing concussion regulations. Current guidelines imply that as long as players sufficiently 'recover' from concussion prior to returning to play, repeat incidence is unproblematic (Partridge and Hall 2014). Concerns relating to CTE are clearly behind calls for a rethink of these assumptions, but an additional and more precautionary layer of regulation might be to restrict the frequency and/or overall number of concussions that can be sustained. Such developments would (currently) be based on questionable scientific knowledge and therefore be, essentially, precautionary. Ultimately, however, they would mainly *shift* the focal point of pressure rather than resolving difficult decisions about who should and should not be 'allowed' to play sport.

Whether taking regulatory control away from sports governing bodies or imposing a reconceptualization of the problems, one overarching barrier to game-related solutions will remain. Specifically, we have seen how the uniquely stringent regulation of concussion injuries (e.g. mandatory removal from play and subsequent period of abstention) creates more pronounced problems for athletes, and disincentives for compliance. But more proscriptive regulation does not necessarily lead to more compliant behaviour, and tighter regulation may even have a negative impact on participants' health as individuals are forced to withdraw from medical supervision. Ethical considerations of player autonomy, and 'first do no harm', will continue to shape game-related solutions.

Cultural change

As a fundamental premise of this book has been that sport's concussion crisis is essentially cultural, it logically follows that cultural change will be necessary to any resolution. There should, however, be no complacency about the ease with which such solutions can be implemented. Cultural change, by definition, is broader in scale and wider in scope than the measures identified so far. Yet if, as noted in Chapter 1, cultural crises entail deep-rooted social conflicts which are usually resolved through the emergence of new cultural formations, this type of change must be our primary consideration.

Chapter 6 charted the many attempts to reduce the incidence of concussion injuries through interventions seeking to modify the behaviour of (particularly) youth athletes and so change the culture of sport. It was noted that these were frequently predicated on psychological assumption. We might, therefore, describe these as micro-cultural changes. However, these programmes are largely ineffective, and while in part they fail because they are initiated in isolation from more macro-oriented cultural change, there is also a fundamental paradox to biomedically designed public awareness campaigns in that they involve attempts to make a group which is believed to be acting 'irrationally' behave in a 'more rational' manner (i.e. in medically prescribed ways). While such programmes could become more rather than less sensitive to the values of the target audience (e.g. developing concussion awareness campaigns that emphasize the deterioration of post–concussion functional performance), the persistence of the 'problematic' behaviours suggests that 'more of the same' is unlikely to lead to major attitudinal shifts.

Ironically, part of the problem these interventions face is the positioning of concussion as a unique form of injury. While this signals the heightened degree of potential risk and therefore the greater level of precaution is justified, it is ultimately counter-productive in that distinct forms of regulation create particular forms of behaviour. Moreover, the 'exceptionalism' of concussion serves to generate research which is likely to enhance the sense of crisis because results cannot be compared to other related behaviours (i.e. the non-reporting of non-concussion injuries). Constructing concussion injuries as so distinct that usual ethical considerations (patient autonomy and confidentiality) should be abandoned inhibits broader *cultural* change in favour of promoting more localized and discrete interventions. The sense of 'crisis' is inherently linked to the idea that there is something fundamentally distinct about head injury. While this cannot be discounted, neither should it be exaggerated.

The call to locate concussion within a more holistic concern about attitudes towards, and the incidence of, sports injury represents the beginning of a more macro-oriented cultural change agenda. Essential to this is a reconsideration of the sport-health ideology. The sport-health ideology leads to a relative lack of questioning about the role of physical education in school curricula, the 'concerted cultivation' of children through extracurricular sports clubs, etc. The social commitment to this ideology obscures the relative danger of sports participation and forces sports organizations to project relatively low levels of potential risk. But a more measured and critical appraisal of the outcomes of sports participation would reduce expectations and thus the apparent contradiction that fuels the crisis. A further consideration is that in conjoining the sport-health ideology with the moral rhetoric of childhood we are left with narratives of concussion which appear to relegate the potential seriousness of the issue for adults. Until we recognize that injuries are widely experienced within the active sports population, and thus (at best) the 'necessary evil' to be balanced against the socially valued aspects of participation, our aspirations for sport will continually exceed the outcomes.

Secondly, our 'reading' of sport must also be revised such that the great and expanding differences between the injury implications of elite and 'ordinary' sport are more explicitly recognized. The commercial imperatives which give rise to the sport celebrity culture work against our recognition of these differences, but sport's concussion crisis will not be resolved while we continue to conflate the incidence and experience of injury in these highly atypical occupations with those of the wider sports playing population. Indicatively, professional soccer players in the UK experience 500 times more workplace injuries than those in the next most dangerous occupation (Hawkins and Fuller 1999). We could, for instance, be much more transparent about the physical toll inflicted by elite sport training regimes and the longer-term holistic health impact on these individuals. In so doing, we might also break the link between these activities and masculine national identity. While people engage with these sporting activities for the enjoyment they bring and the excitement they generate, their construction as totems representing 'our' nation in global 'proxy' wars creates identities largely built on 'imagined' affiliations (Anderson 1983). If those chosen to represent 'us' in our national sports ever really did have a connection with the broader constituency of followers, it has been weakened by the hyper-specialization and commercialization of modern elite sport. Separating out these two very distinct levels of sporting experience would allow us to disaggregate some of the spill-over effects which complicate the concussion crisis. Specifically it would allow us to hold the otherwise contradictory prioritization of 'safety first' or 'first do no harm' for the many and individual sovereignty (where 'informed consent' exists) for the few for whom sport is an occupation.

Of course, the ultimate 'solution' rests on recognizing the interdependence of SRC with a broader and more complex web of social processes, namely developments in relation to medicine and health, the perceived need to protect children, and our concerns about ageing. These are both deeply intertwined with, and fuelled by, sport's concussion crisis. Although fundamentally altering these processes by attending simply to the issues around concussion is overly ambitious, a greater recognition of how the attitudes that stem from these wider considerations influence our approach to SRC will at least help *manage* the crisis. Particularly important is greater reflection on the degree to which we seek to insulate our children from life's inherent risks, our fears over the needs of more elderly and ageing populations living with chronic illnesses (and specifically dementia-related conditions), the contradictions in our expectations for and scepticism about the efficacy of modern medicine, and our expectations of what constitutes 'health'. Each of these factors mediates the way in which we receive and interpret concussion-related evidence from sport. The value of historical study is that it shows us how previous concerns about sporting injuries were 'deeply tied up with ideological, moralistic, religious, and even nationalistic beliefs about the role of youth sports, as well as the country's direction more broadly' (Bachynski 2019: 24). The promise of social science is to deploy these lessons as we seek to ameliorate contemporary concerns.

The problems of invoking cultural change appear to be compounded by our post-truth condition, and the 'most obvious response . . . is to counter misinformation with facts' (Lockie 2017: 1). This is clearly one option for sport's concussion crisis, for, as we have seen, the relatively high degree of scientific uncertainty enables different factions to 'chose' evidence which supports their pre-existing positions and, subsequently, talk past rather than to each other. But the limitation of this approach is that, currently, we see that the representation of 'counter-fact' frequently serves to re-entrench positions and reinforce perceptions of collusion and conspiracy by opponents pursuing their own set of vested interests. The emotive recourse to 'protecting' children is a case in point. While this is undoubtedly an effective tactic in garnering support for a particular position, the lack of empirical substantiation means that it may equally lead to suspicion and distrust, and stronger opposition. Legal and coroner pronouncements (about CTE and SIS) which conflict with the 'consensus' of medical opinion and significantly go beyond the existing evidence hinder the process. An immediate goal must be to stop the escalation of the divisions which create crisis and inhibit resolution.

Recognizing that cultural change is difficult is very different to suggesting that it is a futile exercise. All of these changes (biotechnical and game-related changes included) represent opportunities to enhance the lives of individuals and militate against the harms of taking part in sport. There are real concerns about the consequences of head injury which stem from tangible and observable harms experienced by sporting populations. A multidisciplinary approach is necessary to address a set of issues that impact upon and have drawn in so many different spheres of contemporary society. Through cross-cultural comparison we can begin to cut through the more locally specific and emotive concerns and provide better context through which to understand sport's concussion crisis. But, ultimately, we need to be aware of the broader or global social processes which, in 'coming to a head' in sport's concussion crisis (pun intended), make for a particularly challenging, self-perpetuating, and irresolvable cultural crisis.

References

Anderson, B. (1983), *Imagined Communities: Reflections on the Origin and Spread of Nationalism*. London: Verso.

Bachynski, K. (2019) '"The duty of their elders": doctors, coaches, and the framing of youth football's health risks, 1950s-1960s', *Journal of the History of Medicine and Allied Sciences*, 74(2): 167–191.

Cantu, R. and Hyman, M. (2012) *Concussions and Our Kids*. Boston, MA: Mariner Books.

Carlisle, W. (2018) 'The AFL's concussion problem: is the league running interference on the damage concussion can cause?' www.themonthly.com.au/issue/2018/september/1535724000/wendy-carlisle/afl-s-concussion-problem

Caron, J. and Bloom, G. (2015) 'Ethical issues surrounding concussions and player safety in professional ice hockey', *Neuroethics*, 8: 5–13.

Fuller, S. (2018) *Post-Truth: Knowledge as a Power Game*. London: Anthem Press.

Goldberg, D. (2013) 'Mild traumatic brain injury, the National Football League, and the manufacture of doubt: an ethical, legal, and historical analysis', *Journal of Legal Medicine*, 34(2): 157–191.

Greenhow, A. (2018) *Why the Brain Matters: Regulating Concussion in Australian Sport*. Unpublished PhD thesis, Monash University, Melbourne Australia.

Hawkins, R. and Fuller, C. (1999) 'A prospective epidemiological study of injuries in four English professional football clubs', *British Journal of Sports Medicine*, 33: 196–203.

Lockie, S. (2017) 'Post-truth politics and the social sciences', *Environmental Sociology*, 3(1): 1–5.

Malcolm, D., Sheard, K., and Smith, S. (2004) 'Protected research: sports medicine and rugby injuries', *Sport in Society*, 7(1): 97–110.

Partridge, B. (2014) 'Dazed and confused: sports medicine, conflicts of interest, and concussion management', *Bioethical Inquiry*, 11: 65–74.

Partridge, B. and Hall, W. (2014) 'Repeated head injuries in Australia's collision sports highlight ethical and evidential gaps in concussion management policies', *Neuroethics*, 8(1): 39–45.

Sanchez Garcia, R. and Malcolm, D. (2010) 'De-civilizing, civilizing or informalizing? The international development of mixed martial arts', *International Review of the Sociology of Sport*, 45(1): 1–20.

Sismondo, S. (2017) 'Post-truth?', *Social Studies of Science*, 47(1): 3–6.

Stewart, W., Allinson, K., Al-Sarraj, S. et al. (2019) 'Primum non nocere: a call for balance when reporting CTE', *Lancet Neurology*, 18: 231–232.

Timmermans, S. and Buchbinder, M. (2012) 'Expanded newborn screening: articulating the ontology of diseases with bridging work in the clinic', *Sociology of Health and Illness*, 34(2): 208–220.

INDEX

CPSIA information can be obtained
at www.ICGtesting.com
Printed in the USA
LVHW020722090423
743866LV00018B/221